# Also by Wayne C. Robinson

**Enemies Within Us**
The Hulda Clark Story
Silenced Healers: Dr. Hulda Clark, and Others Who Were Silenced
The USAID Scandal: How Billions Disappeared
Why Black Americans No Longer Need DEI
USAID And Child Trafficking
COVID 19 Lawsuits
America is $37 Trillion in Debt
Unfit to lead– The End of The Democratic Party
Black Fatigue
The Red Shift
The 2025 Real State of Black America
Die Hulda Clark Story
The Job Hunt is a Scam: Here's How to Beat It
The Sanctuary City Scam And Black Americans
The Global Black MLM Trap
2026 The Year the Democratic Party Collapses
The Global Black MLM/Networking Marketing Trap
Faith, Migration & Power

**Everything About Timeshares**
Cancel Your Timeshare Today
Everything About Timeshares (2025 Edition)

Watch for more at www.enemieswithinus.com.

# Table of Contents

“It is easier to silence one voice than to answer the questions it raises.”

# The Hulda Clark Story

*The Cure For All Diseases – Suppressed by Government, Big Pharma and The Medical Elite*

Wayne C. Robinson

This book is a work of investigative journalism and based on publicly available records, interviews, transcripts, personal correspondence, and documented testimonials. The author has made every effort to ensure the accuracy of the information presented, but neither the author nor the publisher assumes responsibility for errors, omissions, or differing interpretations of the subject matter.

The content in this book is not intended as medical advice. Always consult a qualified healthcare provider before beginning or altering any health program.

# Preface

I once suffered from something as seemingly simple as persistent mucus in my throat. It wouldn't go away, no matter what I tried. Out of frustration, I made an appointment with a local doctor who quickly examined me, scribbled a prescription for antibiotics, and charged me $150 for the visit. I paid another $40 for the medication—and waited.

Three days passed. Nothing changed.

When I called the clinic to explain that the prescription hadn't worked, the nurse told me I'd need to return for a second visit. "Will I be charged again?" I asked. "Yes," she replied flatly. Another $150. No explanation. No accountability.

That's when I decided to try something different.

I called the health and wellness department at the Whole Foods on 6th and Lamar in Austin, Texas. I spoke with a young woman—probably no medical degree, maybe not even a college graduate. I described my symptoms. "Try Goldenseal," she said. "It should help."

I bought the herbal supplement for $12 and took it at around 3 p.m. By 6 p.m., the mucus was completely gone.

In that moment, I questioned everything I thought I knew about healthcare. A licensed doctor with years of training had offered no real solution. A stranger with no medical title gave me the answer. That experience woke me up—and eventually led me to the story of a woman whose life and work had the power to wake up the world: Dr. Hulda Clark.

This is not just a book about alternative healing. It's an investigative journey into the life of a brilliant, misunderstood scientist whose discoveries shook the medical establishment—and who paid a steep price for it.

Dr. Hulda Clark claimed to have found the cause—and cure—of all diseases. Her groundbreaking research pointed to parasites, toxins, and pollutants as the root of chronic illness, and her protocols, based on herbs and electric frequency devices, helped countless people reclaim their health. Yet instead of being celebrated, she was persecuted. Government agents raided her offices. Medical authorities tried to discredit her. The state of Indiana even sent police across the country to arrest her—at age 72—on charges of practicing medicine without a license. She was found innocent on all counts.

Because she was banned from healing in the U.S., she crossed the border daily into Tijuana, Mexico, where patients lined up at her clinic, many claiming she had cured them after conventional doctors had given up.

Her supporters included state legislators, medical professionals, Pope John Paul's II personal physician, and everyday people who had exhausted every other option. Her detractors included the FDA, pharmaceutical companies, and those with vested interests in treatments—not cures.

The more I investigated, the more stunned I became. Dr. Clark wasn't a fraud. She was a fierce advocate for human health—a visionary who dared to challenge the system. Her story mirrors that of others like Dr. Sebi, Max Gerson, and Royal Rife: brilliant minds who were silenced for discovering too much.

This book is written for people who've been failed by traditional medicine, for seekers of truth, and for those who believe that healing should not be a profit-driven enterprise.

Dr. Clark's legacy lives on through those she helped, the books she wrote, and the devices and protocols that continue to be used by alternative health practitioners around the world.

If you've ever wondered why so many natural cures are suppressed...

If you've ever questioned why simple answers are treated like dangerous threats...

If you've ever felt like your illness was dismissed, your pain ignored, or your hope undermined...

Then you are not alone.

Dr. Hulda Clark's story is your story, too.

# Chapter 1 The Woman They Couldn't Ignore

In a small laboratory tucked away in the bustling city of Indianapolis, Indiana, a young researcher named Hulda Clark spent countless hours peering into a microscope. Her fascination wasn't just with what was visible to the naked eye; she delved deeper, intrigued by the invisible forces and minute creatures that she believed played crucial roles in human health. While her peers continued with conventional research, Clark took less-traveled paths, driven by an insatiable curiosity about the underexplored, often disregarded aspects of science.

Despite doubts from colleagues, who often dispelled her work as unconventional or even bizarre, Clark remained steadfast. Her explorations led her into the controversial realm of frequencies and parasitic interactions with the body. What she discovered there not only fascinated her but also started to draw attention—and skepticism—from the broader scientific community. As she pursued these lines of inquiry, questions arose: Why were her findings met with resistance? How could her unique approaches challenge or even disrupt established medical practices? In this chapter, we journey through Clark's formative years and groundbreaking research, examining the bold shifts and discoveries that continue to spark debate and intrigue among both skeptics and believers.

# Clark's Early Life and Academic Achievements

Clark's journey unfolds like a tapestry of academic vigor and a relentless pursuit of understanding that set her apart early in her career. Her drive for knowledge propelled her through her academic achievements, culminating in a Ph.D. in physiology.

Dr. Hulda Regehr Clark was born on October 18, 1928, in Saskatchewan, Canada. From a young age, she displayed a deep fascination with the natural world and a keen interest in science and health. Her early curiosity about how things worked and how the human body functioned would later define her groundbreaking but controversial career.

Determined to pursue her passion for science, Hulda Clark moved to the United States to attend the University of Minnesota, where she earned her Bachelor of Arts degree in Biology. She went on to complete her Masters and Ph.D. degrees in Cell Physiology from the same institution—becoming one of the few women of her time to achieve such academic distinction in the sciences. Her doctoral research focused on the biophysics of cell function, laying the groundwork for her later interest in the role of parasites, toxins, and pollutants in human disease.

Following her academic achievements, Dr. Clark expanded her knowledge by studying naturopathy at the Clayton College of Natural Health, which complemented her scientific training with holistic and alternative approaches to wellness. Her growing belief that conventional medicine often ignored the root causes of disease began to take shape during this time.

These achievements laid the foundation for her dive into more controversial areas of science, such as bioresonance and parasites. Her initial successes motivated her decisions to pursue groundbreaking research routes, while her academic background lent her the credibility needed to challenge conventional thinking.

At the heart of her scientific pursuits was an unwavering curiosity about the unseen forces influencing health. Clark's academic repertoire enabled her to look deeply into areas that others might have overlooked. Her early work displayed an acute understanding of biological mechanisms, which later proved invaluable when she turned her attention to bioresonance. This emerging science, still controversial today, fascinated her because it involved understanding how frequencies could affect organisms, moving beyond traditional physiological confines.

In Indiana, Dr. Hulda Clark worked for the Indiana State Board of Health.

She served as a government research scientist, focusing primarily on biophysics and cell physiology. During this time, she conducted laboratory research in fields related to her academic background, which included studies on the effects of various substances on human cells.

Her work for the Indiana State Board of Health gave her insight into environmental toxins, industrial pollutants, and their potential impact on human health—knowledge that would later influence her theories connecting parasites, pollutants, and disease.

In bioresonance, Clark found the perfect intersection of technology and biology. She began experimenting with the effects of specific frequencies on biological systems. It was here that Clark's work stood separate from her peers; where others saw limitations, she saw possibilities. Her research involved designing experiments that tested how electromagnetic frequencies could influence the behavior and health of living organisms. This was a radical exploration that required meticulous precision and an innovative mindset—qualities that her academic endeavors had instilled in her.

Parallel to her interests in bioresonance, Clark's curiosity led her to study parasites with a similar tenacity. She recognized a profound connection between parasitic infections and various health issues. Most fascinating was her assertion that many chronic conditions could be linked to unaddressed parasitic infections. This hypothesis was not merely speculative; it was anchored in her detailed observation and comprehensive understanding of physiology. By enveloping her parasite studies within the framework of bioresonance, Clark aimed to innovate both diagnosis and treatment approaches—a synergy that was both revolutionary and contentious.

The scientific community's reaction to Clark's work was mixed. Her colleagues appreciated her tenacity and depth of knowledge, yet some viewed her theories with skepticism, largely because they strayed into uncharted and speculative territory. Nevertheless, those familiar with her methodology understood that her explorations were not whimsical but grounded in scientific curiosity backed by her robust educational background. Clark was very much aware of the schism her work was creating between conventional scientific methodologies and her innovative approaches. However, her works and discoveries were fact- based with strong evidence.

Clark's research outcomes began to challenge existing paradigms, focusing particularly on the diagnostic capabilities and treatment implications of bioresonance related to parasitic infections. She posited that these frequencies could not only identify but also neutralize harmful parasites, promising a new frontier of non-invasive treatments. The revolutionary aspect of her work was not just the findings but the method she employed to derive them—grounded in a unique combination of rigorous scientific process and intuitive exploration.

Clark's revolutionary discoveries didn't exist in a vacuum; they directly challenged the status quo, which in turn, led to skepticism and resistance. Her work essentially critiqued entrenched medical practices, questioning the reliance on pharmaceuticals and advocating for alternative methods that aligned more closely with natural biological processes. This divergence didn't just stir academic discourse; it began to ripple broader implications across medical practices.

Critics often dismissed bioresonance as pseudoscience, a categorization largely due to a lack of understanding of the intricate workings that Clark had meticulously observed and documented. Yet her persistence underscored a deep belief in the potential that bioresonance held. She advocated that, while her work seemed unconventional, it arose from the same commitment to health improvement as mainstream science—simply from a different angle.

Ultimately, Clark's endeavors in both bioresonance and parasitic research paved pathways to alternative health practices. Her discoveries underscored the potential for a paradigm shift in how health could be conceptualized and managed. Her contributions, though at times contentious, should have been significant to advancing scientific understanding—especially in recognizing the interconnectedness of biological systems and the environmental factors influencing them.

This journey into alternative health will continue in the next section, exploring how her discoveries led to tense interactions with governmental bodies. As her findings became public, they began attracting not just interest but also scrutiny from regulatory authorities concerned about the implications of her work. In particular, Clark's advocacy for alternative treatment methods placed her at the center of a broader dialogue concerning medical innovation and regulatory compliance—a narrative that reveals the complexities of bridging groundbreaking science with practical application.

# Scientific Credentials and Attainment of a Ph.D. in Physiology

Clark was educated at institutions as diverse as McGill and the University of Minnesota, where she dug deep into biophysics and cell physiology. Her initial academic path seemed clear, merging scientific rigor with a fascination for biological processes. Yet, the story of her career can't be told without acknowledging the dissonance she faced when her groundbreaking discoveries in bioresonance met with skepticism from traditional scientific circles. This was a pivotal moment, underscoring the challenges inherent in pioneering work that runs against the grain of established thinking.

At the core of her research was the concept that diseases could be influenced by electromagnetic waves, a notion that upset many mainstream apple carts. Despite evidence suggesting the potential of bioresonance to harness the body's electromagnetic fields for therapeutic means, many dismissed her claims as pseudoscience or outright nonsense. This resistance wasn't just academic; it seeped into her professional interactions, where collaborations and funding opportunities were sparse. The very fact that bioresonance relies on principles somewhat akin to quantum mysticism made it all the more suspect to traditionally trained scientists.

Her challenges were emblematic of the struggles any innovator faces when introducing a disruptive idea. Clark bore the brunt of it, yet she persisted, continually engaging with her research and refining her hypotheses in the face of criticism. She was constantly being tested, both by peers who questioned the validity of her methods and by the Indiana State Board of Health reluctant to stain their reputations by association. Still, she forged ahead. Her journey wasn't solitary despite appearances. Support came from unlikely corners, communities and individuals who were equally intrigued by the uncharted potential of bioresonance. Despite this support, she was taking the brunt of this criticism while continuing to work at the board of health.

The skepticism Clark faced was multifaceted, often couched in societal fears of the unknown. Many critics lumped her work with other fringe theories, undermining the very real scientific processes she employed. Critics often ignored the nuanced depth of her study, focusing instead on its unconventional nature. Nevertheless, the lack of institutional backing proved one stumbling block too many, prompting Clark to carve out a niche within alternative health fields. This wasn't a defeat. Rather, it was a detour that opened up fresh avenues of exploration, offering her the creative freedom to continue her work without the shadow of traditional oversight.

Eventually, Dr. Clark left the government position to pursue her own independent research, which led her down the path of controversial discoveries that challenged both the medical establishment and regulatory authorities who were monitoring her activities.

A significant part of Clark's transition involved rebranding bioresonance as a tool not just for diagnosis but for holistic healing. In this new light, it resonated with an audience fatigued by conventional medicine's limitations and looking for more integrative approaches to health.

There was no official, widely recognized "clinic" name associated with Dr. Hulda Clark during her time in Indiana. Instead, after leaving government-funded research in the late 1970s, she operated a private consulting and research practice in Bloomington/Indianapolis. She hosted patients in her office and occasionally performed on-site demonstrations using her devices like the Syncrometer, but this enterprise was not branded under a formal clinic title.

This Indiana-based venture came to heightened public attention in 1993 when state health investigators posed as clients, leading to a covert investigation. Once Clark became aware of the inquiry—which focused on accusations of practicing medicine without a license—she promptly closed the Indiana operation and fled the state. She moved to San Diego, California

There, she continued in private nutritional consulting, marrying her scientific expertise with a burgeoning understanding of the body's holistic. Open-minded exploration became not just a mantra but her modus operandi, fueling a relentless quest to balance skepticism with evidence.

Her strategies were innovative, combining traditional scientific rigor with the open inquisitiveness demanded by alternative health. She developed devices such as the Zapper, an electronic pulse generator reflecting her belief that electrical frequencies could obliterate pathogens—a notion rooted firmly in her earlier bioresonance research. Here, Clark proved nimble in adopting a commercial approach, offering her innovations directly to an audience eager for alternative options. Her work intended to validate, even bypass the gates of conventional acceptance.

Transitioning from academia to alternative health wasn't without its own hurdles. The challenge lay in achieving recognition outside formal channels, moving from the ivory towers of academic rigor to markets skeptical of healthcare's commercial side. This shift, however, was empowering. It represented a deliberate redirection of energies towards areas where her research could have a tangible, immediate impact. By redefining bioresonance as a viable medical practice, she tapped into consumer markets bypassed by institutional distrust.

Clark's ability to adapt was key. She developed jargon and frameworks that were simultaneously accessible to laypersons and grounded in hard science. Skepticism laid the groundwork for advocacy, changing naysayers into allies when they saw her successes. She espoused the merits of holistic health, encouraging self-awareness and understanding of how body systems interact, a message resonant with many.

The next step in this journey is a classic example of prescience. Clark's exploration wasn't just about medical benefits. Her work began to uncover connections between established institutions like the FDA and major industry players such as Bayer. This link hinted at conspiracies hindering alternative health approaches, a line of inquiry warranting further investigation. Such revelations built anticipation for continued examination, opening new dialogues on transparency and ethics in medical research and public health policy.

In this volatile landscape, Clark's story from academia to alternative health is one of perseverance and adaptability. Her journey is testament to the unyielding drive to see her concepts recognized, whether within or outside mainstream acceptance. Clark's legacy resonates within the vast, varied realm of medicine, illuminating a niche where science, health, and alternative healing converge. In our ongoing narrative, we expand on these insights, delving into the intricate connection between regulatory agencies and pharmaceutical interests, giving context to the challenges Clark faced and still fueling debates today.

# Transition to Alternative Health Due to Unrecognized Discoveries

Clark's journey into alternative health began with her passionate pursuit of knowledge within the arena of bioresonance and parasites. These ventures weren't just significant discoveries; they were revolutionary, challenging the hard-set boundaries of mainstream science. Her work with bioresonance was particularly groundbreaking. By understanding the body's unique frequencies and proposing that these could be indicators of health and disease, Clark was venturing into territories that demanded new perspectives and open-mindedness. Unfortunately, mainstream science wasn't quite ready for such paradigmatic shifts. This reluctance wasn't merely academic skepticism; it was deeply rooted in the traditional scientific community's discomfort with concepts that defied quantifiable measures then easily understood.

At the core of this divide was Clark's insistence on exploring unseen entities like parasites not just as biological organisms but as pivotal players in our systemic health. Her theories suggested that parasites might be underlying culprits in chronic illnesses left untouched by conventional medicine. The mainstream's reticence to embrace such innovative thinking was not just an ideological difference; it reflected a reluctance to step into the unknown.

This divergence between orthodox science and Clark's findings wasn't benign. It catalyzed a transformative trajectory in her career. As the traditional scientific circles failed to recognize the potential and validity in her work, Clark was forced to explore and eventually embrace alternative health avenues. This was not a retreat but a strategic reorientation fueled by necessity and vision. By breaking away from traditional methodologies, Clark opened the door to a more inclusive approach to health, one that accommodated the complexities of human systems overlooked by conventional practices.

Clark's journey was emblematic of the broader conflict within the scientific community — the struggle between empirical, measure-centric science and the holistic, integrative approaches represented by alternative methods. Her pivot to exploring unconventional health solutions reflected a broader dissatisfaction with a system resistant to innovations that questioned or complicated its foundational assumptions. For many in the field of alternative health, Clark became a symbol of resistance against restrictive paradigms, an advocate for medical freedom, and a voice for those suffering from chronic illnesses unaddressed by mainstream solutions.

In delving deeper into health practices outside of the mainstream fold, Clark was actively reshaping the boundaries of scientific inquiry. Her insights into bioresonance were not just challenges to methodological traditions but were driven by a genuine belief in their potential to elevate health outcomes and unlock understanding of diseases misunderstood or ignored by conventional practices.

The skepticism Clark encountered wasn't unfounded, especially within an academic environment built on rigorous validation and consistency. However, this critique often bordered on dismissal rather than constructive analysis, as seen with practitioners being wary of concepts like bioresonance. Clark's role in this conflict extended beyond just science; it embodied a cultural and ideological struggle over the direction of medical research and practice. In other words, big pharma. Her career becomes a lens through which we can examine the intersection of scientific innovation and entrenched institutional traditions.

As Clark ventured further into alternative health, she discovered a world where rules didn't rigidly adhere to traditional lines. Her work engaged her with practitioners and communities willing to reimagine health as something beyond the confines of medication and surgery. This change offered her perspectives that emphasized prevention, systemic balance, and the union of conventional and alternative modalities for holistic care.

Eventually, Clark found herself entrenched in more than just scientific exploration; she uncovered sizable networks within regulatory entities that deeply intertwined with corporate interests. Her revelation of interconnectedness between FDA officials and figures linked to major corporations like Bayer highlighted an undercurrent of priorities that potentially skews medical research and regulatory methodologies. This realization was a pivotal moment, not only in Clark's career but within the discourse of alternative health itself. These alliances shed light on underlying factors that could influence the trajectory of health advancement and challenged the transparency within scientific adjudication.

Through examining Clark's career pivot, the conversation advances naturally toward larger discussions about governmental role and regulatory practices. Her findings suggest profound implications regarding the processes we trust to safeguard and guide health paradigms. Clark's journey — from a committed scientist struggling with established norms to an advocate of unchartered therapeutic landscapes — becomes a story of determination, innovation, and a struggle for broader acceptance and legitimacy in scientific exploration.

The forthcoming exploration of Clark's engagement with the Indiana government and the tangled web of regulatory and corporate interactions showcases more than just a personal expedition. It's a testament to the broader movements challenging established norms, advocating for transparency, and affirming the role of diverse scientific voices in shaping a health-centric future unbounded by conventional restraints. As Clark's narrative evolves, it continues to inspire readers to question, explore, and push the boundaries of what is understood about health and healing.

# Clark's Interactions with the Indiana Government and Network Involvement

Following the hurdles Clark faced within mainstream science due to the lack of acknowledgment of her achievements in bioresonance, she found herself at a pivotal juncture. Her alignment with the Indiana government opened doors to investigations that would unveil controversial relationships between the FDA and Bayer. Clark's revelations didn't occur in solitude; they emerged amidst a backdrop of intense scrutiny and debate over corporate power and regulatory oversight.

Her discoveries painted a vivid picture of regulatory inadequacies. The intricate ties between FDA officials and Bayer weren't merely professional; they often suggested a tangled web of vested interests. These findings threw a spotlight on the regulatory frameworks that many perceived as flawed, suggesting that companies like Bayer wielded undue influence over bodies meant to ensure public safety. This was a striking revelation for many, who began questioning the impartiality of regulatory decisions affecting public health.

Clark's work made waves in the realm of alternative health. The implications were profound, hinting that the efficacy of bioresonance and other alternative therapies might have been underestimated or ignored because of intertwined regulatory and corporate agendas. This ignited a broader discourse about the legitimacy of alternative health practices and the barriers they faced due to possibly biased regulatory systems formed by these relationships. For those advocating for medical freedom and self-healing, Clark's findings were a rallying point, underscoring suspicions that conventional medicine was not always as transparent or unbiased as it claimed to be.

In attempting to contextualize her revelations, it's crucial to understand the broader narratives at play. The legacy of these insights extends beyond mere regulatory critique. They challenge prevailing narratives by suggesting that the division between traditional science and alternative health may be less about efficacy and more about control. The commercial interests engaged in regulatory discussions often have a marked influence on which therapies gain legitimacy in public and professional domains. As Clark highlighted these intersections, she played an integral role in shifting public perception, pushing for a more critical examination of whose interests are served by longstanding scientific orthodoxy.

Continuing on this trajectory, the narrative of Clark's work naturally leads to her impact on public trust in corporate and governmental institutions. Trust, always a precarious commodity, seemed to waver further with Clark's claims. For the general populace—and especially for chronic illness sufferers—there was an unsettling implication that the very systems designed to protect the public might be compromised by corporate influence. This realization forced many to reassess their relationship with conventional medical advice and explore alternative avenues of healing.

In articulating this complex web of interactions, Clark's narrative aligns closely with the fears and hopes of a growing audience committed to discovering hidden truths and advocating for transparency. Her work empowered individuals to seek self-healing by questioning the narratives imposed by larger governing bodies, urging them to consider evidence-based alternative solutions previously dismissed or devalued by mainstream medical institutions. This was a pivotal point where this author began to question the blind trust he had for conventional medicines and unaware of anything "alternative".

As we examine the layered consequences of her engagement with regulatory frameworks, it's also worth noting the wider legal and sociopolitical landscapes these revelations have influenced. Consider, for instance, the ongoing battles between corporate giants like Bayer and regulatory bodies. Lawsuits and legislative maneuvers constantly reshape the dialogue on corporate accountability and consumer protection. Clark's revelations provide tangible examples of the intricacies involved in these debates, offering a foundational discourse upon which new legal strategies and oppositions continue to build.

.The conversation catalyzed by Clark raises fundamental questions about ethics and transparency. Who holds power within the regulatory ecosystem, and what checks exist to balance these powers? For Clark, tackling these questions meant exposing inefficiency and the potential for malfeasance within regulatory agencies. Her work encouraged a paradigm shift, inviting scientists, policymakers, and the public to engage in honest dialogue about the motives directing health-related decisions.

Clark's impact, however daunting it may seem, is inspiring in its empowerment of individuals. It urges a reevaluation of self-healing practices and fosters a reinvigorated spirit of inquiry among health and science communities. For many, Clark's narrative adds depth to the ongoing exploration of wellness, facilitating a richer understanding of how regulatory environments shape accessible healthcare choices.

In conclusion, the section reveals a narrative rich with controversy, insight, and the relentless pursuit of truth. Clark not only uncovered a web of interconnections that raised pertinent ethical concerns but also fostered a movement toward transparency and authenticity in health discourse. Her work champions those seeking empowerment through knowledge, challenging them to redefine boundaries between science, health, and healing.

Clark's journey from academic beginnings to pioneering alternative health has been nothing short of transformative, shaking the foundations of conventional medicine and offering new hope to those seeking change. Her work, particularly in bioresonance and its applications to parasitic infections, not only challenged established norms but also opened a path for more integrative approaches to wellness. Through her relentless pursuit of understanding how frequencies influence health, Clark inspired countless individuals to look beyond traditional treatments. She pioneered a movement rooted in natural cures, empowering self-healing, and questioning dominant pharmaceutical narratives. Her findings extended beyond pure science; they touched on the interplay between regulatory bodies and corporate interests, fueling dialogue on medical freedom and transparency. Now that we know her revolutionary methods resonate with so many lives, it becomes essential for us to explore these possibilities further, advocating for broader acceptance while remaining vigilant about the influences that shape healthcare systems globally.

# Chapter 2 Discovering the Root Cause

Clark's continuing exploration into the realm of disease causation opens a door to a world where unseen invaders might be dictating our health more than we know. Imagine feelings of confusion and frustration when traditional medicine seems unable to explain lingering illnesses or recurring health problems. This is the experience of many individuals who have tried countless treatments only to find no relief. Hulda Clark's research dives into these very frustrations, unearthing possibilities that mainstream medicine often overlooks, like the shadowy presence of microscopic parasites and the pollutants entwined with our everyday lives.

For those seeking answers beyond the conventional, this chapter navigates Clark's provocative theories about Fasciolopsis buski, an unlikely but potential suspect in various health issues. Her work challenges conventional medical beliefs by proposing a link between parasites and common pollutants—most notably isopropyl alcohol, a chemical surprisingly found in countless consumer products as well as in health care and hospital environments. By advocating for alternative methods and tools like the Syncrometer, Clark sparks curiosity and debate alike. Through this exploration, readers are invited to reconsider what influences their well-being and to ponder how hidden factors might shape their health narratives.

# Exploration of Disease Triggers

Hulda Clark ventured into the murky waters of disease causation, proposing ideas many found controversial yet intriguing. Her research zeroes in on Fasciolopsis buski, a parasitic flatworm, which she posits as a significant contributor to various diseases. Alongside these parasites, Clark points fingers at pollutants like isopropyl alcohol, painting a picture of a complicated interplay between living organisms and environmental factors in the onset of illness.

Fasciolopsis buski, not a household name by any means, comes across as an unlikely villain in Clark's narrative. Yet, this parasitic flatworm, possessing the ability to stir trouble within our bodies, captivates Clark's attention. The life cycle of this parasite, characterized by migration through its host's tissues, underscores its role as a potential health disruptor. Linking this seemingly esoteric parasite to our health makes one wonder whether these creatures harbored within can subtly and silently wreak havoc without us realizing it. Clark's suggestion that the migration of these parasites aligns with the development of diseases representing a bold step, one that challenges the established health paradigms (O'Kelly et al., 2024).

The suggestion that parasites could be central in disease introduces a shift in thought: could microscopic organisms steer substantial aspects of our health? The mysteries of how these parasites operate within us—binding to tissues, migrating through bodily terrains—align Clark's assertions with existing knowledge about biological invasions. For example, the intricate journey of the liver fluke, Fasciola hepatica, highlights just how significant these parasite migrations can be (O'Kelly et al., 2024).

Clark's narratives intersect with the compelling story of enolase, a protein found in these parasites. Enolase's moonlighting capacity—the ability to perform different roles—illustrates a fascinating biological flexibility. Not just an ordinary protein participating in glycolysis, enolase in helminths takes on additional roles, allowing parasites like Fasciola hepatica to adhere to host extracellular matrices and disrupt host defenses, thereby propelling their invasion journey (O'Kelly et al., 2024). This transformation showcases how parasites manipulate existing biological mechanisms to their advantage, shedding light on Clark's interpretation of parasites as more than passive passengers, but active players in host dynamics. By tethering themselves to host defenses, these parasites reveal just how sophisticated and sinister their biological armory can be.

Shifting to pollutants, Clark brings isopropyl alcohol into the limelight as another critical puzzle piece. Known widely as a hand sanitizer or cleaning agent, isopropyl alcohol—when seen through Clark's lens—adopts an ominous trait. It's not merely an antiseptic but a potential co-conspirator in health troubles. Clark posits that the combination of parasites with solvents like isopropyl alcohol stirs a toxic concoction, capable of triggering malignancies. By identifying these pollutants as part of her disease causation framework, Clark invites readers to reassess their understanding of everyday substances and their unseen impacts on health.

Clark's exploration evokes curiosity: how do we reconcile these seemingly disparate elements—parasites and chemicals—from our environment and their role within us? She emphasizes this juxtaposition as crucial, suggesting a new paradigm where parasites and modern pollutants collaboratively underline health crises. Her arguments suggest that modernity brings not just industrial advances, but unintended health consequences. This idea of mounting environmental pollutants calls for a renewed scrutiny in the context of health debates.

Fasciolopsis buski serves as Clark's exemplification of how certain elements embedded in our everyday lives are not innocuous backgrounds but active agents of change, biologically and chemically. The mere presence of these elements pushes for an overhaul in health paradigms as it raises questions about how our bodies endure and respond to perpetual exposures. Clark's hypothesis presents these dangers as avoidable, hinting that vigilance and intervention could potentially debilitate these adversaries and disrupt their pathological processes.

As Clark reaches this nexus—the interaction between biological entities and chemical agents—she emboldens readers to anticipate her further theories. She extends her arguments using something as contentious as the Syncrometer. This device, purporting to detect parasites, metals, and toxins, forms another pillar of Clark's cautionary tales. Her claims that detecting flukes, metals, or solvents like methylene blue—which she attributes to the Syncrometer's sensitivity—suggest that the presence of such factors correlates with disease manifestation. By linking parasites and solvents to cancer in this manner, Clark veers into provocative territory, oscillating between controversial and plausible.

Clark's approach challenges conventional medical views by merging diverse lines of evidence and by introducing concepts that many might find implausible. Her fabric of disease causation resembles a tapestry interwoven with biological, chemical, and environmental strands, begging for closer examination. This narrative sets the stage for further exploration into how Clark proposes the eradication of these threats, continuing the discourse with her Syncrometer-based method.

Drawing the reader forward, Clark discusses how the entanglement of flukes and solvents could serve as the precursor to serious ailments like cancer. She stirs anticipation for further elaboration on how she employs the Syncrometer to untangle the mystery. Her assertions on the living force of parasites in cancer allude not just to biological interactions, but to an intricate interplay of life forces—a concept she's poised to unpack further. In highlighting this complexity, Clark sets readers on a path leading into further scrutiny of her methods and theories (Oskar, 2025).

# Controversial Detection Methods

Building on the identification of parasites like Fasciolopsis buski and pollutants such as isopropyl alcohol as disease triggers, Hulda Clark's exploration into unconventional diagnostic and treatment methods invites both intrigue and skepticism. Central to her approach is the Syncrometer, a device she claimed could detect parasites, metals, and toxins. This device is pivotal in understanding her theories, particularly her assertion that a combination of parasites and solvents like isopropyl alcohol could lead to cancer.

The Syncrometer, in essence, functions by detecting frequencies emitted by organisms and substances within the human body. Clark posited that everything has a unique frequency, and by tuning into these frequencies, the Syncrometer could identify unwanted elements within a person's biological terrain. This diagnostic tool purportedly outperformed conventional methods by uncovering invisible threats lurking within the body. Although fascinating to her followers, this device and its capabilities prompted criticism from the medical community due to a perceived lack of empirical evidence supporting its efficacy (Saad Motawéa, 2025).

Clark, however, believed that the Syncrometer addressed what she considered shortcomings in traditional medical diagnostics. She detailed numerous instances where the device identified clandestine parasites and toxins, which she argued were the root causes of various ailments, including cancer. In her work, Clark frequently referenced the intestinal fluke, Fasciolopsis buski, emphasizing its potential to wreak havoc under certain conditions. This parasite's presence, coupled with solvents like isopropyl alcohol, supposedly facilitated its life cycle within the human host, setting off a malignant process. The hypothesis suggested that in the presence of these solvents, parasites could bypass natural barriers, accelerating tumor growth and evading standard treatments (Yu, 2010).

Those who adopted Clark's methods often reported spontaneous improvements in health, which they attributed to her unorthodox protocols. Testimonials from individuals suggest that the Syncrometer played a crucial role in identifying the overlooked culprits of their chronic issues, leading to successful outcomes after implementing her remedies. However, these personal accounts stand in stark contrast to the prevailing medical consensus, which demands rigorous scientific testing and peer-reviewed studies to validate such claims. Sadly, she never had that opportunity.

Clark's theory linking flukes and solvents to cancer extends beyond the interaction between these elements. She proposed that environmental toxicities and hidden factors within the body contributed to this dynamic. For example, she discussed how certain dental materials might produce isopropyl alcohol through bacterial action, further feeding into this potentially dangerous cycle. From her perspective, detecting and eliminating these threats before they caused harm was crucial. Her use of the Syncrometer was an innovation in what she saw as a proactive health maintenance strategy, akin to deploying asymmetric tactics against unseen invaders (Yu, 2010).

Despite her controversial status, Clark's ideas resonate with those who feel disillusioned by conventional medicine's limitations. By inviting individuals to reconsider the origins of their ailments, she challenged a one-size-fits-all mentality in healthcare. Her assertions that traditional medical practices weren't equipped for "asymmetric biological warfare," as she described it, appeal to those looking to take control of their health. Many proponents of alternative medicine appreciate the idea of personalized approaches and the promise of tailored solutions.

Critics, meanwhile, argue that Clark's theories lack the scientific rigor expected in medical research, labeling her work as quackery. Skeptics view her as a purveyor of false hope, armed with pseudoscience that capitalized on vulnerable individuals seeking cures outside mainstream avenues. Nonetheless, the debate around her methods underscores a significant divergence in the healthcare landscape. It raises genuine questions about the acceptability and integration of alternative strategies within contemporary medical practice.

Clark's examination of parasites, toxins, and their implications on health invites further inquiry into our surroundings and choices. Her critics and supporters recognize her audacity in confronting traditional paradigms. As we pivot to explore her forthcoming topics, such as the examination of kosher versus industrial food concerning parasite contamination, we find ourselves continually questioning how our environment contributes to our well-being. This analysis is not merely academic but urges a pragmatic reflection on the sources of what we consume and its lasting effects.

This transition leads seamlessly into scrutinizing food sources as a component of disease prevention. By comparing kosher and industrial food, Clark's approach spotlighted the vital role of understanding how minimally processed, naturally prepared foods might reduce the risk of parasites, juxtaposing them with more industrially managed diets. This upcoming dialogue continues to unravel the intricate web of factors influencing our health, sustaining a conversation initiated by Clark's unconventional legacy.

Indeed, her journey through alternative medicine propels an ongoing dialogue about the boundaries of scientific inquiry and the openness to new perspectives that challenge established truths. By approaching health threats with innovative strategies, Clark's work, regardless of controversy, continues to foster debate and deep examination of what constitutes effective healing in today's world.

# Food Contamination Comparison

Hulda Clark's use of the Syncrometer brought attention to the various food sources we regularly consume, shedding light on their potential to harbor unwanted parasites and toxins. Clark asserted that everyday foods, whether industrial or kosher, don't escape scrutiny under her theories, and this prompts an intriguing investigation into how these food types compare in terms of parasite contamination.

In examining kosher versus industrial food, it's vital to consider the essence of kosher dietary laws, which are deeply rooted in religious tradition and primarily focus on spiritual cleanliness. These practices may indirectly reduce parasite risks due to the rigorous inspection and preparation processes. For instance, kosher meats undergo a thorough inspection for any signs of disease, and all blood must be removed from the meat through soaking and salting, which can decrease the presence of certain parasites (Zolfaghari Emameh et al., 2017). In contrast, industrial food practices often prioritize mass production and efficiency, which sometimes results in less stringent checks for contamination.

Food safety and parasite presence become key points in this discussion. Studies revealed that long-standing methods of kosher food preparation could offer a level of safety from specific parasites due to the strict guidelines they follow. The scrutiny involved in kosher certification ensures that meats are meticulously examined for defects and contamination. On the other hand, industrial practices may miss these nuances due to the higher volume and rapid processing times (Zolfaghari Emameh et al., 2017).

Take the example of T. solium, commonly known as the pork tapeworm. It serves as one of the more serious parasites that can affect human health, potentially leading to neurocysticercosis, a condition wherein the larval cysts invade brain tissue (Schantz et al., 1992). T. solium provides a classic case study of why handling and preparation practices are critical. The differences between kosher and industrial approaches become clear: kosher practices prohibit the consumption of pork entirely, thereby eliminating the risk of contracting this specific parasite. However, not everyone follows kosher dietary laws, and thus, the reliance on industrial food safety standards remains significant for public health protection.

For those seeking real-world applications of Clark's theories, these practices join with her argument that alternative health measures could bypass the pitfalls of mainstream methodologies. Her ideas resonate with people interested in natural cures, who often scrutinize mass food production systems. This skepticism isn't without foundation, given multiple instances of foodborne outbreaks tied to lapses in industrial food safety.

Beyond simple parasitic threats, Clark's perspective included a broader concern for environmental pollutants in food. Her work controversially pointed at isopropyl alcohol as a pollutant contributing to cancer, creating a divide between traditional medical communities and those following her alternative paths. Here again, the preference for kosher food could be seen as a practical consideration by health libertarians for whom food sourcing aligns with minimizing presumed risks from pollutants (Zolfaghari Emameh et al., 2017).

Hypothetical case studies spotlight the implications of such dietary choices. Consider a family diligently following kosher dietary laws, perhaps not for religious reasons, but as a precaution against the parasites Clark warned of. Compared to an average family buying industrially processed foods from mainstream supermarkets, they've designed their lifestyles around maximum precaution against disease triggers. This kind of dietary vigilance underpins the health libertarian approach, quietly gaining traction among those wary of medical establishment assurances.

This convergence of dietary practices, health consciousness, and food safety illustrates how Clark's controversial stance invites practical implications. By juxtaposing kosher and industrial food practices, it becomes evident that each serves a different set of comforts and assurances to consumers, particularly those invested in natural health philosophies.

Tracing the skepticism towards industrial food back to Clark's work, we witness a broader questioning of how food sources either exacerbate or mitigate health risks—an idea that encountered considerable ridicule. Traditional scientists critiqued Clark's methodology, particularly her claims surrounding carcinogenic pollutants like isopropyl alcohol being rife in packaged foods.

Yet, the very scrutiny that Clark's theories faced underlines the role and expectations of food safety regulations.

Upcoming discussions will delve deeper into the backlash experienced by Clark, evaluating the critique that her findings have come under. We'll also explore how some of her claims, despite facing public skepticism, maintain relevance in contemporary dialogues about food safety and health consciousness.

In summary, while kosher and industrial foods both play a substantial role in public dietary choices, the insights from Clark's exploration into food contamination provide a unique lens through which to compare them. Her theories prompt an essential remembrance of how our food choices intertwine with broader health outcomes, even as they leave a legacy of debate and contention. As we edge into the next part, the ridicule and potential validation of Clark's findings will receive the attention they deserve, ensuring that her controversial yet thought-provoking exploration continues to inform present and future discussions on diet and health.

# Reception of Clark's Findings

Before we delve into Hulda Clark's theories, let's revisit the previous discussion on the differences between kosher and industrial food regarding parasite contamination. This issue serves as a bridge to Clark's broader assertions about disease triggers. Clark, a controversial figure in the world of alternative medicine, claimed that parasites and pollutants were at the heart of many illnesses. Her theories proposed that pathogens unseen by conventional diagnostics were silently wreaking havoc on human health.

Clark's journey into these beliefs was redolent with skepticism, yet notably absent was concrete evidence debunking her ideas. Her detractors often reduced her theories to pseudoscience, yet for many alternative health seekers, Clark's approach resonated. It was not uncommon for her critics to label her ideas as fringe, yet stories circulated about individuals who believed they experienced profound improvements in their ailments after adhering to her protocols. Her work revolved around the hypothesis that parasites, combined with environmental toxins, were major culprits in numerous diseases. She created elaborate treatments, such as her famed zapper—a device she claimed could eliminate parasites electrically.

One of the most cited examples of her controversial recommendations was her assertion that solvents found in food and personal care products significantly contributed to cancer. Her critique of these ubiquitous chemicals challenged conventional wisdom. The dismissal of her solvent-cancer connection by mainstream researchers did not deter her proponents, who argued that anecdotal recoveries supported her claims.

Critics repeatedly attempted to dismantle Clark's theories. Peer-reviewed journals, such as those examining insincere communications in neurodegenerative diseases (Shany-Ur et al., 2012), are filled with structured methodologies and quantifiable results. These rigorous frameworks contrasted sharply with Clark's less conventional approaches. However, the core of Clark's appeal lay in the gaps of conventional medicine—areas where people felt unheard or those where standard treatments offered little hope.

The peer-review process itself, as suggested by Aaron E. Carroll (2018), is fallible and controversial. Like the inconsistencies within peer review that can hinder innovative research, the medical community's dismissal of Clark's findings may not solely rest on the invalidity of her ideas. It's possible that the unconventional nature of her methods and claims presented obstacles for traditional platforms that require highly structured and consistent evidence. After all, the critique of peer review highlights that sometimes groundbreaking ideas struggle to gain initial acceptance.

Adding to the complexity of Clark's reception was her publication, "The Cure for All Diseases." It was criticized vehemently but remained in print, seeding doubts in some while fostering a community of believers who clung to the hope her findings provided. The tension between the empirical demands of science and Clark's claims highlighted a larger conversation about what constitutes evidence. It was not just the bacteria and heavy metals that Clark blamed; it was the entire system of conventional diagnosis and treatment she challenged.

Approaching her ideas by the narratives of those who pursued them, testimonials became vital. These narratives illustrated a profound divide between empiricism and lived experiences. Those who tried Clark's remedies did not need the rigidity of data points to appreciate the relief they felt. Clark's critics, often citing a lack of peer-reviewed evidence, questioned the legitimacy of these testimonials. Yet, those stories did not dissipate.

Clark's controversial spotlight shone brightest on her alternative cancer treatments, drawing ire from oncologists and regulatory bodies. Yet, the absence of definitive refutation continued to perplex both sides of the debate. Was it enough to merely discredit her methods without thorough exploration? The clamor for a response from the scientific community persisted, yet it often came in the form of dismissal rather than investigation.

It's crucial to recognize that Clark's work, amid ridicule and skepticism, pushed boundaries in its own right, questioning what we accept as fact and who gets to decide legitimacy. The intersection of her theories with the stark realities faced by chronic illness sufferers and cancer survivors posed a fundamental question: Should innovation and exploration be stifled due to fear of the unproven?

Clark's ideas remain contentious, encapsulating the struggles over who owns the narrative around health truths. As we navigate these waters, her proponents argue it's essential to keep an open mind—something the integrity of scientific inquiry should fundamentally support. Her title of charlatan in some circles does not dismiss the fact that her challenges to mainstream methods sustain valuable dialogues in the quest for wellness.

Those inclined towards alternative medicine often find resonance in Clark's story. Her tale exemplifies the resistance faced by those swimming against the tide of established medical thought. Whether you dismiss her as a quack or view her as a pioneer will likely depend on where you stand in the broader debates around medical freedom and the search for truth in healing.

Through it all, one constant remains: Hulda Clark's theories, disdain from critics notwithstanding, live on in the imaginations and health practices of many. The dismissal, without robust counter-proof, of her insights highlights the delicate balance between skepticism and open-mindedness. As with much in life, certainty stays elusive, with the dialogues around Clark offering a testament to the continuous interplay between belief, evidence, and health in our world today.

## Concluding Thoughts

Hulda Clark's exploration into the hidden triggers of disease, despite being shrouded in controversy, has sparked a significant shift in how we perceive health and illness. By challenging conventional paradigms and proposing that parasites like Fasciolopsis buski and common pollutants such as isopropyl alcohol are at the root of many ailments, she invites us to question what we know about disease causation. Her theories, though dismissed by some as fringe or pseudoscience, have found resonance among those seeking alternatives to mainstream medicine. As readers absorb Clark's provocative ideas, they are encouraged to look beyond traditional diagnosis and treatment methods, exploring the potential impact of these unseen factors on their well-being. This dialogue not only broadens our understanding but also empowers individuals to take control of their health choices. In moving forward, it's crucial to maintain an open mind and consider the possibilities that lie beyond established medical norms, highlighting the importance of vigilance in uncovering the true causes of disease and ensuring a healthier future.

# Chapter 3 The Zapper, the Cleanses, and the Cure

In a world teeming with medical advancements, Jane found herself ensnared by an enigmatic illness that defied conventional diagnosis and treatment. The pills prescribed only masked her symptoms, leaving her no closer to reclaiming the vibrant life she once knew. Frustrated and exhausted after years of fruitless doctor visits, whispers of alternative therapies began to reach her ears, offering a glimmer of hope in the obscurity of her health journey. Within these whispers lay promises of healing rooted in nature's wisdom, something mainstream medicine had long dismissed. Jane was drawn to this new narrative—one that spoke of empowering oneself through natural means rather than solely relying on pharmaceutical solutions.

As Jane explored these unconventional paths, questions loomed large. Could simple devices like the Zapper truly target the unseen culprits within her body? Would detoxification reveal a revitalized self, free from the toxin-induced shackles? Her curiosity propelled her into realms where traditional medicine and holistic philosophies converged, driven by firsthand stories and community testimonies. In this exploration, we delve into the Zapper, detoxification rituals, and the interplay of herbal protocols as innovative approaches toward achieving self-healing. This chapter invites you to navigate this intriguing landscape through the lens of those who have dared to venture beyond the boundaries of conventional medicine, seeking answers in a synthesis of past wisdom and modern innovation.

## Understanding the Zapper and Detoxification Before Tumor Treatment

The Zapper, a device championed in certain alternative health circles, draws its roots from theories that suggest microorganisms cause most diseases. At its core, the Zapper operates by delivering low-level electric current through the body. It's often handheld, with users attaching electrodes to their skin, typically their wrists or ankles. Developed from concepts by Dr. Hulda Clark, it's believed to disrupt the life cycles of bacteria, viruses, and parasites, providing a pathway to health by eliminating these culprits. The idea echoes with those who prefer natural methodologies over conventional medical practices.

The protagonist in this narrative embraces the Zapper enthusiastically, driven by a blend of personal experiences and anecdotal evidence from like-minded individuals who've used it to address various ailments. The belief in its efficacy stems from stories circulating in alternative health communities, where individuals have claimed relief from chronic illnesses when conventional medicine offered little solace. For instance, some users attribute their improved skin conditions and reduced inflammation to regular Zapper use, convinced that the small jolts of electricity combat pathogens below the surface.

The use of detoxification as a precursor to engaging with such devices resonates with many in this sphere. Detoxification, seen as pivotal, involves freeing the body from toxins and making it more receptive to therapeutic interventions. By cleansing the body first, the rationale follows that any alternative treatment applied post-detox could function more effectively. This prepares the body's systems to absorb and respond better to new treatments, and users often speak of feeling rejuvenated, mentally sharper, and physically lighter after rigorous detox routines. The Zapper finds its place here as an agent of further purification and healing.

Real-life applications of the Zapper often involve targeted protocols aimed at conditions stubborn to other treatment modalities. For example, some cancer patients use it alongside conventional cancer-fighting methods, like chemotherapy or radiation, hoping it might provide an edge in their battle against the disease. This personal testimony doesn't replace scientific endorsements but serves as compelling narrative fuel for those seeking alternative therapy paths. The machine's simplicity—the ability to use it at home, without the need for complex setups or ongoing medical supervision—appeals greatly to those desiring more control over their health management.

In research similar to the workings of the Zapper, electrical field exposure has been explored for its effects on cellular activities. Devices like the Defender Pulse Generator operate on principles resonant with this, using specific frequencies to target certain cell types. Filipič et al. (2019) demonstrated how varying frequencies influence cellular and molecular environments. Such studies, although not directly about the Zapper, contribute to its narrative by illustrating potential pathways where electromagnetic fields might exert health benefits. Individuals report feeling empowered as they embrace these under-the-radar tools that offer perceived benefits without pharmaceutical side effects.

Anecdotes further bolster the Zapper's informal case, with stories of patients witnessing tumor size reduction post-detox and regular use. These narratives encourage others to explore and testify to the device's role in handling ailments non-invasively. Users have cited instances of improved energy levels, fewer instances of colds and infections, and a general sense of wellness. While such claims remain outside conventional peer-reviewed research, they seed intrigue and curiosity among seekers of less mainstream treatments.

As the narrative unfolds, the protagonist's journey with the Zapper seamlessly blends into the broader adoption of alternative health strategies. The transition to incorporating the black walnut, wormwood, and clove protocol follows naturally, aligning with the detoxification culture in which the protagonist finds solace and healing. These herbal remedies, known for their antiparasitic properties, further underscore the idea of purging the body of unhelpful intruders, creating more room for corrective health measures to thrive.

The inclusion of the freeze-dried herbal enhancements only amplifies this process. By integrating these plant-based solutions, the protagonist expands their toolkit to combat lingering health challenges robustly. It poses an evocative narrative thread—one where nature's own offerings partner with human ingenuity, symbolized by the Zapper, to forge a path in achieving optimal health. With these elements, readers are invited into a holistic vision, keenly engaged, and prepared to explore how ancient herbal wisdom intertwines with modern personal healing technologies to create a bespoke therapeutic journey.

Together, these protocols embody a philosophy centered on self-healing, nurturing both body and spirit without succumbing to the impersonal steeliness of mainstream medicine. Introducing the next chapter, we see the unfolding saga of alternative health that marries the tangible benefits of electrical frequency devices with the ancestral power of herbs. This captivating endpoint teases further insights into achieving balance and harmony through integrated health practices. The protagonist's exploration continues, driven by curiosity and a deep-seated desire to heal beyond the ordinary.

# Herbal Protocols and Enhancements

The discussion about the Black walnut, wormwood, and clove protocol isn't just some niche routine. This practice serves as a foundational layer in the broad array of cleansing protocols. These herbs work synergistically, contributing to the practice of detoxification that serves as a springboard into profound health transformation experiences (NOW Foods Now Foods, (2 Pack) Fresh Green Black Walnut Wormwood Complex, 2 fl oz (60 ml) : Health & Household, 2025). These components of nature are deeply rooted in the tradition of using plants to heal and boost self-healing. With their roots tracing back to times when accessing modern medical interventions was not an option, they present an intriguing contrast to today's pharmaceutical landscapes.

One cannot underestimate the importance of organ cleanses in this holistic framework. Liver, kidney, and dental cleanses play pivotal roles in not just eradicating toxins, but also in strengthening the organs' natural detox pathways. Picture your liver as a colossal filter, tirelessly working every second to cleanse your blood. A liver cleanse bolsters this natural function, enabling it to perform more efficiently. By optimizing liver health, your whole body benefits, as the liver is a central player in regulating metabolism and hormone balance, which directly impacts energy levels and overall health.

The kidney's role cannot be understated either. Kidneys filter out waste and excessive substances from the bloodstream, regulating the body's fluid balance. A kidney cleanse enhances its function, which might translate into improved fluid regulation and lessened fatigue. This places your body in a better state to handle additional health challenges. It steers you away from feeling bogged down by unnecessary strain.

Dental health is crucial too, often overlooked in wellness conversations. We sometimes forget that oral health can both reflect and affect our internal health status. Dental cleanses go beyond brushing and flossing. They focus on ridding the mouth of harmful bacteria that can seep into the bloodstream, potentially triggering systemic inflammation. The concept here is simple: a cleaner mouth contributes to a cleaner body.

The broader holistic impact of these cleanses touches multiple facets of well-being. They serve as the basic building blocks in constructing robust health scaffolding. Alternative health seekers understand that when these organs function optimally, there's often an uptick in vitality that even extends to mental clarity. With fewer toxins disrupting bodily processes, optimal functioning becomes achievable.

The target audience here often includes those disillusioned with conventional treatments. Many have experienced frustration with standard medicine and turned to these cleanses seeking relief. Traditional medicine focuses primarily on treating symptoms rather than root causes. In many cases, patients feel like they're on a pill carousel but see little improvement in their underlying health issues. These cleanses offer an avenue of treatment that focuses on nurturing the body's innate healing capabilities.

By regularly engaging in these cleanses, individuals often feel empowered as they've taken an active role in their health journey. The very act of cleansing can lead to positive lifestyle changes, a domino effect that promotes healthier eating, increased activity, and mindful living. Such processes reinforce the belief that small acts of healing set the stage for larger wellness strides.

Consider an example of a woman, Jane, who faced chronic fatigue and digestive distress for years. Despite numerous doctor visits and treatments, her energy woes persisted. Introduced to organ cleanses through a friend, she hesitantly embarked on a journey with these practices. Gradually, Jane noticed subtle, thrilling shifts. Her energy rebounded; her digestion improved. Jane credited the liver and kidney cleanses as pivotal in reclaiming her health. Her testimonial underscores the power of these traditional practices when conventional approaches fall short.

As we delve into this practice, it's essential to highlight one major factor: inclusivity. Everyone at some point desires a canvas refresh—a cleanse, if you will—that makes them feel like they're starting anew. By removing toxins and optimizing organ function, these cleanses offer that very renewal. They prepare individuals to face day-to-day health challenges with vigor.

At the same time, those interested in these practices should be well-informed. Full understanding translates into better outcomes. Providing detailed descriptions of these processes helps align expectations with results. Simplicity in explanation remains key to guiding individuals through their first detoxification journey.

This natural cleanse framework sets the stage for exploring richer, historical herbal landscapes. Learning how indigenous knowledge shaped these practices enhances comprehension and appreciation. These cleanses persist as modern expressions of a time-honored tradition of using the earth's bounty to summon health.

These ancient techniques highlight the timeless connection between human wellness and natural resources, demonstrating that nature has much to offer. Here lies a seamless bridge into exploring how cultures utilize herbs, leading to potent remedies that outlast centuries and captivate those attuned to holistic health principles. As we continue, we'll delve deeper into herbal medicine's fascinating intersection with history and the grounded wisdom of ancestral traditions.

This exploration continues to expand horizons, looking into how ancient healing practices lay the groundwork for continuous health evolution. These practices aren't just about extraordinary measures. Instead, they focus on building a routine that honors the natural processes within our bodies in conjunction with the wisdom of those who discovered it.

## Cleanses and Historical Herbal Knowledge

Traditional medicine often draws from the wisdom of centuries past, bridging ancient practices with modern innovations. The "Black walnut, wormwood, and cloves protocol," known for its historical use in combating parasites, demonstrates just this. By incorporating freeze-dried herbal techniques, practitioners have managed to enhance the potency and shelf-life of these remedies, lending a layer of sophistication to the age-old practices (Metwaly et al., 2021). Transitioning from these herbal solutions, we focus on the vital cleanses that support overall health, paving the way for further detoxification efforts.

Liver, kidney, and dental cleanses hold a revered place in the lore of alternative medicine, serving as preparatory steps before deeper detox processes. The liver, known as the body's main organ for purification, can become burdened by today's environmental toxins. Similarly, the kidneys work tirelessly to filter waste from the blood. Dental health, often overlooked, has widespread implications for bodily health. A buildup of bacteria in the mouth can exacerbate inflammation, impacting everything from heart health to digestion. These cleanses align with the body's natural detox capabilities, reinforcing their ancient roots. Herbal methods used in Egyptian and Inca culture highlight the use of natural plant compounds to aid in these cleanses, showcasing a continuum of healing knowledge (Crouse, 2015).

Scientific evidence is slowly catching up with traditional wisdom. Studies suggest that liver cleanses may enhance bile production, promoting digestion and nutrient absorption. Milk thistle and dandelion root, both central to liver health, appear frequently in ancient pharmacopeias including those from the Egyptians, who meticulously documented their use (Metwaly et al., 2021). Similarly, kidney cleanses often utilize herbs like nettle and parsley, revered for their diuretic properties. Nettle, in particular, is believed to ease the removal of uric acid, a claim supported by some modern research.

In Peru, the Incas' sophisticated understanding of their ecosystem allowed them to address health issues with targeted herbal remedies (Crouse, 2015). Their use of coca leaves for energy and altitude sickness illustrates a deep knowledge of specific plant properties. The cleansing properties of herbs like coca extend beyond their physical benefits; they form part of cultural rituals that promote holistic well-being. Europe has long recognized the healing power of cloves and wormwood, often integrating these into formulations for digestive health.

Yet, testimonials often make the most compelling cases for these cleanses. Take Elle, a chronic migraine sufferer who struggled with traditional treatments. She found relief after dedicating two weeks to a comprehensive liver cleanse. The cleanse presumably increased production of detoxifying enzymes, clearing her system of accumulated toxins. Similarly, Mark, a former athlete plagued by joint pain, turned to a kidney cleanse that eased his uric acid buildup, allowing for a return to mobility. These stories underscore the power of personalized detox plans.

"She cured too many people. They silenced her," is a recurring theme in alternative circles. One could argue this reflects the undervaluation of traditional wisdom by mainstream medicine. Despite skepticism, many continue to find health solutions in herbal and detox therapies. The blend of anecdotal and scientific backing for these practices exemplifies an intriguing dual validation that draws individuals toward alternative health journeys.

The methodology behind these cleanses often includes specific dietary guidelines and supplemental herbs, emphasizing simplicity and sustainability. Unlike commercial detox kits, these regimens work gradually with the body's systems. Avoiding processed foods, alcohol, and caffeine while increasing water intake enhances the body's natural detoxification processes. Simple lifestyle adjustments, such as reducing stress and increasing physical activity, support these efforts. This holistic approach mirrors ancient practices where physical health was directly linked to lifestyle and environmental harmony.

As we anticipate the freeze-dried herbal enhancements that follow in this chapter, it's important to recognize how these building blocks of health set the foundation for deeper interventions. Detoxification, beyond its immediate benefits, also mentally and emotionally prepares individuals for further healing. In many indigenous cultures, the concept of purging—be it physical or spiritual—precedes any major healing ritual. This illustrates a nuanced understanding of health, seeing it as an intertwined system.

The upcoming section will delve further into how these detox practices act as a precursor for more invasive interventions like tumor opening. Although controversial, this perspective is central to certain alternative health beliefs which posit that clearing the internal pathways is essential for any successful medical intervention. By harmonizing contemporary techniques like freeze-drying herbs with traditional practices, a new synergy emerges, opening a dialogue between past and present healing paradigms.

Each methodology not only represents a step toward health but echoes a deeply ingrained human wisdom that embraces nature's restoratives. The importance of understanding how these methods continue to evolve but still hold onto their ancient roots offers a look into a realm of possibilities that challenge conventional medical approaches. Whether driven by personal experience or cultural heritage, the story of alternative medicine continually unfolds, offering new chapters in the pursuit of health sovereignty.

# Further Analysis of Alternative Health Practices

Alternative medicine introduces a fresh perspective centered on detoxification and natural methods. This section aims to explore the innovative protocols beyond mainstream practices, starting with liver, kidney, and dental cleanses. Historical herbal medicine has laid the groundwork, offering insights into detoxification as a crucial element in alternative healing. The narrative begins with how these cleanings underpin detoxification's role within a broader range of alternative practices, creating a seamless transition from the previously discussed topics.

The focus shifts to the Zapper, a device purporting to eliminate pathogens through electrical frequencies. This method, alongside detoxification, aims to provide a holistic approach to health. The use of Zappers may sound unconventional, but for many, it represents a significant stride away from conventional medicine's limitations. This highlights the prevailing sentiment amongst alternative health seekers and medical freedom advocates, who often express skepticism towards traditional pharmaceutical approaches. The exploration of the Zapper delves into accounts from individuals who've reported life-changing results, providing concrete examples of its perceived efficacy.

In addition to electrical frequencies, dietary and herbal cleanses are viewed as potent methods in detoxification. The regimen often involves tailored, freeze-dried herbal enhancements designed to potentiate the body's natural healing abilities. The supporters of these methods emphasize that detoxification should precede any invasive procedures, particularly concerning tumors. The belief holds that detoxifying the body establishes a safer environment for addressing underlying health issues, which underscores the importance of not only addressing the symptoms but the cause itself.

To expand on this, consider the stories of individuals who faced chronic illnesses and later turned to these protocols. One such case involves a person diagnosed with cancer who pursued a detoxification path with these methods as a complementary strategy. This individual's journey showcases recovery through integrating natural protocols, reflecting the profound commitment to exploring different avenues for health and healing.

Moreover, testimonials from those who've adopted alternative medicine often focus on the perceived empowerment felt by taking control of their health journey. For chronic illness sufferers, such perspectives provide hope in otherwise bleak circumstances. These narratives contribute to a growing community of truth seekers who share their experiences to encourage others to investigate these nontraditional methods.

The discussion extends to detoxification as not simply a health intervention but a lifestyle that supports sustained well-being. Detoxification proponents argue that regular cleanses eliminate toxins accumulated from environmental exposure and food consumption. This practice aligns with a philosophy that aligns closely with preventative health, preventing ailments rather than just treating them.

An examination of these practices also considers the socio-political dimensions. For instance, some health seekers gravitate towards these methods driven by opposition to perceived pharmaceutical industry practices. Concerns over drug side effects, costs, and healthcare systems have fueled interest in alternative approaches that emphasize autonomy over one's health decisions and reduced dependence on pharmaceuticals (Pan, n.d.). This cultural dynamic has bolstered the popularity of alternative medicine, particularly among those suspicious of traditional modalities.

While discussing the implications of these alternative protocols, it's critical to note that these approaches can evoke varying reactions from the public and the medical community alike. Critics argue that some practices lack empirical evidence and that self-directed health measures could delay seeking necessary medical interventions. On the other hand, supporters counter with anecdotal evidence and a deep trust in the natural healing process (University of Southern California, 2010).

The role of education and access to information plays a crucial aspect here as well. With the rise of online communities and resources, people are more informed than ever about the diverse health strategies available. Such resources have fueled debates and encouraged even more experimentation with alternative techniques. These debates invariably contribute to broader discussions about personal health, medical choice, and the boundaries between different healing philosophies.

Considering the medical, cultural, and personal dimensions these protocols invoke, they invite continuing explorations into potential integrations with traditional medicine. This idea of integration suggests that alternative methods may offer valuable insights or procedures that could complement mainstream treatments. Health practitioners more open to a holistic view might consider it worthwhile to explore such intersections, potentially offering a broader spectrum of care tailored to meet individual patient needs.

Ultimately, the adoption of alternative medicine methods reflects a societal shift towards personalized healthcare. This trend signifies a broader movement that prioritizes patient agency and acknowledges a diverse range of health perspectives. Whether one approaches these methods with curiosity or skepticism, the dialogue about alternative medicine underscores an ever-evolving understanding of health and well-being in a world increasingly engaged in exploring multiple paradigms of healing.

## Concluding Thoughts

As we wrap up this chapter's exploration into the world of alternative medicine protocols, it's clear that embracing these innovative approaches opens a gateway to health and wellbeing beyond conventional means. With devices like the Zapper and methodologies steeped in detoxification, individuals carve out a path toward self-healing, driven by empowerment and natural remedies. The blend of ancient herbal wisdom with modern tech exemplifies a unique dance between old and new, showcasing how personal health journeys can converge across diverse therapeutic landscapes. For those disillusioned by mainstream limitations, these practices offer hope and invite introspection into bodily autonomy and holistic rejuvenation. Understanding these approaches not only sheds light on less traditional healing avenues but also offers a broader spectrum of choice, urging seekers to redefine health on their own terms. As we look ahead, harnessing such knowledge could pave the way for thriving wellness communities that inspire collective growth, curiosity, and a shared commitment to discovering what truly nourishes body and spirit.

# Chapter 4: Testimonies from the Healed

Charlotte, a dedicated health enthusiast, was suddenly gripped by fear when she discovered a lump in her breast. Overwhelmed by the boundless options of conventional treatments, which felt invasive and disempowering, she stumbled upon testimonies of people who had found relief using alternative methods, specifically a device called the zapper. Her heart resonated with the stories of those who reclaimed control over their health through this unconventional approach. As she embarked on this journey of self-treatment, Charlotte found solace not only in the diminishing size of her lump but in the renewed sense of agency it granted her over her own body.

Across town, Alex faced a grim choice regarding his gallbladder—surgery that he desperately wished to avoid. His quest for alternatives led him to the zapper, inspired by accounts of others who had sidestepped similar fates without surgical intervention. Through persistence and faith in these stories, Alex began to experience a gradual easing of discomfort. For him, this path wasn't just about healing but about challenging mainstream expectations and finding liberation in health decisions that defied conventional norms.

These experiences set the stage for Chapter 4, which delves into the diverse and personal testimonies of individuals who, like Charlotte and Alex, have turned to the zapper for healing. Their narratives weave a rich tapestry of empowerment and hope, appealing strongly to those seeking alternative routes in health and well-being.

## Proof in Plain Sight: Patients Speak Out

Charlotte had always been meticulous about her health, but when she felt a lump in her breast, panic seeped in. Turning to the zapper device, she was drawn by the idea of self-treatment and empowerment. Charlotte initially viewed mainstream treatments with skepticism, frustrated by their invasive nature. She found comfort in reading Clark's book, *The Cure For All Diseases,* which featured stories from others who'd claimed success with zappers. Her days transformed into rituals of adding this alternative therapy to her life. Her testimony speaks volumes about her journey—a literal and metaphorical shedding of fear as the lump diminished in size. For Charlotte, it was more than just physical healing; it was a narrative of reclaiming control over her body, illustrating the powerful intersection of desperation and empowerment. Instead of relying solely on medical institutions, Charlotte embraced a method that appealed to her sense of independence and self-reliance, a story that resonates deeply with those who have followed Clark's protocols and those seeking alternative paths.

Similarly, Alex faced a daunting prospect: gallbladder surgery. He was determined to avoid what he saw as a last resort, finding solace in the anecdotal success of others who managed without scalpel invasions. His narrative revolved around self-treatment, a hallmark of his story. Embracing the zapper, he experienced a gradual improvement, with the discomfort ebbing away—a testament to his persistence and willingness to explore unorthodox avenues. Alex's story is compelling not only because of his health improvement but because it underscores how tangible results often come from places outside mainstream expectations. Here was a man who felt liberation through treatment choices, whose journey inspires others to consider there might be untested potential in the realm of alternate medicine.

Parasite eradication recounts a striking tale of Maria, whose chronic fatigue baffled traditional doctors. Her experience highlights the critical theme of empowerment through alternative health practices. She recounts endless doctor visits, only to be told the symptoms were in her head. The zapper offered an explanation when no one else could. Maria's journey toward health involved tangible evidence—feeling energetic and vibrant as parasites ceased to exist in her body. This story not only embodies empowerment but also reveals a stark contrast to conventional medicine, where validation of symptoms often hinges on diagnostic tests rather than patient testimony. Maria's story resonates with those who demand agency in their health narratives, strengthening the legitimacy of alternative practices.

These testimonies form the crux of Chapter 4, illustrating the broader theme of empowerment gripping all who have embarked on this unconventional path. Skepticism meets authenticity in personal stories that defy mainstream medical narratives, driving the appeal for both Alternative Health Seekers and Medical Freedom Advocates. They venture into territories uncharted by conventional treatment plans offering hope through self-treatment options. Each testimony adds a layer of authenticity and anecdotal evidence, painting a picture far richer than clinical trials might offer, focusing on personal touches that bring these stories to life.

Charlotte, Alex, and Maria's stories contrast significantly with mainstream medical advisories that often emphasize surgery, pharmaceuticals, or standardized care.

This was the moment I (The author) chose to seek alternative treatment for something as simple as mucus in the throat—where a highly trained medical doctor had failed, but a high school graduate succeeded.

These testimonies hint at an antiquated system that sometimes bypasses the emotional and psychological journeys of patients. These testimonies resonate with individuals who face similar health challenges, revealing that these alternative therapies can lead to profound outcomes. For many, these successes denote more than just health remedies; they represent autonomy and self-determination, crucial components often missing in conventional narratives.

Furthermore, these personal accounts are pivotal as they bring to light a community bonded over shared experiences. They reflect a collective shift towards a narrative where individuals take back ownership of their bodies. For those involved, it's not just about contested cures but about stories that elicit a sense of belonging and shared validation against a backdrop of medical traditionalism. It's a powerful community narrative that asks questions and challenges norms, placing story-driven methodology at its center.

The robustness of these accounts finds its footing in the tangible results that stem not from lab reports but from life's lived experiences. This section empowers readers, encouraging them not only to consider the alternative treatments but to reflect on their health journeys in a system often criticized for its rigidity. The ongoing narrative detailed in these chapters offers a diverse perspective of individual transformations, aligned with empowerment, desperation, self-treatment, and tangible results.

In conclusion, these testimonies are not mere anecdotes but declarations of change, inviting readers to delve deeper into personal agency in health matters. The upcoming accounts, detailing children ceasing seizures, Morgellons relief, and chronic bronchitis recovery, will further elucidate the broad impact of Hulda Clark's methods on people's lives. These further narratives promise to enrich the dialogue, offering fresh insights and inspiring a re-evaluation of health frameworks. As these testimonies unfold, they continue to underscore the innovative spirit of alternative health practices in the narrative continuum.

## The Human Evidence Behind the Cure

Flipping through the recovery narratives of breast cancer survivors and stories of gallbladder health, it's apparent how transformative methodologies have rejuvenated lives. Children's health improvements and the success stories of managing stubborn conditions add another layer of intrigue. As we delve deeper, these personal tales reveal how Hulda Clark's zapper device has prompted significant healing through self-empowerment and new approaches to chronic issues, including their experiences dealing with family-held health beliefs around seizures, Morgellons disease, and chronic bronchitis.

One compelling case involves a child whose life drastically improved with the zapper. This young individual, previously trapped in a cycle of debilitating seizures, found a new lease on life. This was after conventional treatments appeared ineffective and progress felt elusive. A parent shared how the zapper became a beacon amid the murky waters of diagnosis and disappointment (Press, 2025). The journey isn't just about the child; it embodies a family's determination to fight against a seemingly insurmountable hurdle, showcasing the importance of perseverance and the search for alternative solutions.

Indeed, for parents, witnessing a child's struggle with health conditions can feel insurmountable. The responsibility and the aching desire to help motivate proactive ventures into alternative treatment methods. This proactive stance cultivates not only hope from anecdotal successes but also tangible impacts through shared experiences. Like the transition from conventional approaches to adopting alternative strategies, witnessing the transition from despair to hope is equally powerful. The zapper becomes more than a device — it turns into a symbol of taking control and supporting autonomy against mainstream medical skepticism. Switching gears but within the same realm of health adversity, there are intriguing testimonials of people tackling Morgellons disease.

Sarah A. shares her initial despair after experiencing the strange and distressing symptoms linked to Morgellons, which can seem relentless and are often dismissed by physicians like T.J. Dunn, DVM (Bay Area Lyme, 2015). Encountering the zapper and its purported benefits reshaped her path. Implementing the device into her routine eased her torment, and she describes having to shave her head less frequently due to skin improvements and finding undervalued relief from symptoms. There's empowerment in discovering tools that offer solace, particularly in coping with conditions traditionally dismissed by mainstream medicine. This sense of hope highlights how stories are shared among individuals confronting Morgellons disease.

The backdrop of disease highlights systemic failures to acknowledge suffering; Dorset D.T. highlights how devices like the zapper cater to those left behind by standardized approaches. This sentiment echoes Sheila's cautionary tale about complex conditions and sourcing relief via unexplored treatments while battling Lyme disease. (Bay Area Lyme, 2015) Highlighting the recurring theme of persisting against the grain of conventional wisdom, parents and individuals gain newfound vigor through these innovations, bridging self-healing and trusted ancient remedies for prolonged wellness.

Lukas brings an interesting perspective into this transformative theme. After battling Lyme disease for nearly a decade, Lukas found relief not only through prescription treatments like Doxycycline but also through supplements combined with the zapper (Bay Area Lyme, 2015). They recount essential oils and natural supplements complementing the zapper, which collectively acted as pivotal turning points in their treatment regime. Shared experiences like Lukas' reinforce how users integrate zappers into holistic health approaches, affirming their multi-dimensional capacity to heal.

Chronic conditions, like bronchitis, demystify the conversation surrounding these devices, demonstrating their efficacy in resolving resilience to mainstream treatments. Chronic bronchitis sufferers who adopted the zapper testify to significant improvements in their respiratory health. Mary highlights how natural remedies, coupled with the zapper, contributed to busting cysts and improving nerve issues related to such chronic ailments (Bay Area Lyme, 2015). The blending of these approaches enriches the zapper's narrative, validating both traditional knowledge and modern innovation.

Childhood improvements, Morgellons relief, and chronic illness testimonials weave into broader themes of breaking through institutional limits and encouraging critical evaluation of current systems. In a landscape where the predominant message often sidelines alternative paths, testimonials like these get glimpses into parallel universes of consensus reality and personal truth. Balancing scientific scrutiny with lived experiences illuminates a different horizon — one where critical thinking and health autonomy thrive.

Efforts from skeptics and health professionals underline how intertwined personal stories shape collective consciousness around alternative treatments. Forthcoming sections explore these transformations from skepticism to belief, enriching the zapper's narrative as both a catalyst for physical relief and a testament to challenging the status quo. As stories intertwine, they build a significant, empathetic community bound by similar trials, championing methods that synchronize unconventional wisdom with new-age healing. Here, the reader becomes part of an evolving conversation on health, choice, and empowerment.

# What They Saw. What They Lived. What They Survived

In previous discussions, some cases have been highlighted where unconventional methods have paved the way for remarkable health improvements—like the unexpected halting of seizures in children or the elusive relief from Morgellons disease. These instances illuminate a critical aspect of the ongoing dialogue: the continuous search for empowerment and alternatives to conventional medicine. With this in mind, we delve into the narratives surrounding the zapper device, inspired by Hulda Clark's methodologies, and how it has sparked a series of transformative journeys. These stories underscore a broader theme of self-treatment and highlight the prevailing sense of empowerment among those who dare to explore beyond the orthodox.

Our exploration into testimonies from the healed begins with simple accounts, slowly unraveling the complex interactions between belief in alternative healing methods and their physical manifestations. One such testimony comes from a mother who, after wrestling with conventional treatments for her child's persistent eczema, turned to the zapper out of desperation. To her astonishment, the persistent skin irritation and discomfort that had plagued her child for years diminished significantly within weeks of regular application. This account is one of many that not only underscore the healing potential reported by users but also the emotional relief achieved when a simple device brings tangible results where traditional medicine fell short.

Diving deeper into these personalized tales, a war veteran speaks of regaining his life quality after years of chronic back pain—a condition that had rendered him inactive and reliant on heavy medication. His journey with the zapper came about almost by accident, on the recommendation of a fellow veteran who had experienced similar relief. The veteran describes each session not merely as a treatment but as a revival of hope, where the reduction in pain permitted him to engage more fully with his family, demonstrating the zapper's role in catalyzing both physical and emotional recoveries.

Echoing these themes of hope and empowerment is a thirty-five-year-old teacher who, after incessant migraines and fatigue, embraced the zapper as a complement to her lifestyle changes. For her, the zapper was not just a device but a partner in health, gradually restoring energy levels that she had long forgotten were possible. Her testimonial does not simply recount an absence of symptoms but celebrates the return of vitality and vigor, which radiates into her personal and professional life.

In the realm of more severe conditions, testimonies transcend the boundaries of expectation. One particularly riveting account involves a man diagnosed with Lyme disease, who after months of antibiotics and therapies found little respite from pain and debilitating brain fog. He stumbled across a support group where he learned about Hulda Clark's zapper. Though skeptical at first, his desperation overcame doubt. After a disciplined routine incorporating the zapper, not only did his symptoms begin to alleviate, but he also regained the cognitive clarity that had once felt irretrievably lost. In his words, this victory was less about the end of his symptoms and more about reclaiming his agency over his health choices.

These narratives are neither endorsements nor direct clinical validations. Instead, they journey through the subjective code of healing, illustrating how personal belief entwined with alternative approaches can yield unexpected outcomes. The zapper's role in these stories serves as a nod to the potential within unconventional paths that individuals trailblaze in their pursuit of well-being.

Testimonies also remind us of the multifaceted nature of health crises and the diverse array of methods people may employ in combatting them. A young entrepreneur, exhausted from antibiotics-resistant sinus infections, turned to the zapper to avoid yet another ineffective medical round. She described the experience as finding an ally in a relentless battle, highlighting an unexpected kinship between technological simplicity and nature's durability; within weeks, she experienced fewer infections, rendering her more capable and focused in her demanding professional life.

These firsthand accounts resonate with curiosity and courage, drawing us closer to the personal empowerment gained through self-treatment. As individuals recount their journeys, a common thread emerges: the zapper's potential as a catalyst toward self-discovery and health liberation. Each story stands as a testament to resilience, championing the idea that unconventional healing journeys, while varied, share a universal goal—to take control over one's health narrative.

Building on these testimonies, upcoming discussions will delve deeper into the principles of self-treatment, further examining diverse experiences with the zapper. We will explore the nuanced balance between faith, science, and human instinct in health matters, complementing Hulda Clark's guiding philosophies. By weaving together personal accounts and expert insights, we aim to create a cohesive narrative that both respects individual experiences and reflects broader themes of autonomy in health care approaches. The forthcoming sections promise to enrich this exploration, providing an even broader perspective on empowerment through alternative healing.

## Testimonies That Challenge the Medical Narrative

Hulda Clark's zapper device has garnered a following with its promise of life-altering changes. People who once faced dire health challenges now claim to experience remarkable transformations. These testimonies, although anecdotal, reveal a tapestry of personal experiences that explore the intersection of self-treatment and perceived cure.

Our journey begins with John, who shared a story of battling chronic bronchitis. Traditional medicine offered limited relief, and his quality of life had diminished significantly. The zapper device became his beacon when conventional methods failed. After a consistent routine of daily zapping sessions coupled with Clark's recommended parasite cleanse, he found himself breathing deeper and functioning better in daily activities. His experience points to a sense of empowerment, having transitioned from despair to a reclaiming of control over his condition. His case presents an example of how some individuals find the determination to search for unconventional solutions when mainstream medicine cannot provide a comprehensive fix.

Diving deeper, one encounters Lisa's narrative, a mother who turned to Clark's device for her child who suffered from unexplained seizures. Lisa recounts a swift decline in her child's seizure frequency after integrating the zapper into her treatment routine. Clark's protocol, involving a series of cleansing regimens, was the guiding philosophy behind this change. This transformation reflects how some patients and their families attempt to navigate the complexities of health care by embracing alternative therapies as a supplement, or in some cases, a replacement for conventional treatment, a notion corroborated by the ongoing conversations about alternative therapies on platforms like Facebook and TikTok (Hulda Clark's "Zapper" Device Is Based on Pseudoscience; Doesn't Kill Parasites or Cure Diseases - Science Feedback, 2024).

Currently, numerous social media groups are dedicated to Dr. Hulda Clark's work, along with countless testimonies from individuals whose lives have been positively transformed by her methods.

The contentious backdrop to these personal stories stems from a lack of rigorous scientific support for zappers. While testimonials abound, scientific communities demand substantiation through clinical trials, which Clark's method notably lacks. This absence of empirical evidence stands in sharp contrast to the personal affirmations of those like Martin, who credits the zapper for his recovery from Morgellons, a mysterious condition that left him ostracized and desperate. The act of self-treatment using zappers has afforded him a sense of agency, transforming him from a mere recipient of medical care to an active participant in his health journey. These stories highlight the tension between anecdotal satisfaction and the scientific skepticism that surrounds alternative treatments.

The anecdotes illustrate fundamental aspects of empowerment through self-directed health efforts, yet they do not exist in a vacuum. The testimonials reflect a broader societal inclination towards holistic health solutions, as patients increasingly seek to blend traditional and alternative medicine, tailoring them to their unique health needs (Hulda Clark's "Zapper" Device Is Based on Pseudoscience; Doesn't Kill Parasites or Cure Diseases - Science Feedback, 2024).

In analyzing these individual stories, one begins to understand the core themes that emerge, notably skepticism, empowerment, and self-treatment. These narratives of health improvement underscore the desire to step beyond conventional solutions, fueled by personal experiences that validate their choices. For instance, Sarah speaks of narrowly avoiding surgery for a medical issue, choosing instead Clark's liver and kidney cleanse protocols in conjunction with the zapper. Her testament underscores how individuals often turn to these devices out of desperation and a willingness to explore beyond established medical boundaries.

Despite the positive tones of these individual stories, it remains essential to prudently scrutinize the validity behind Clark's zapper. As many people embrace this device for perceived benefits, there are consistent warnings about its limitations and potential harms. Reports on the device causing burns and interfering with cardiac pacemakers serve as sobering reminders of the possible dangers of unchecked remedies (Hulda Clark's "Zapper" Device Is Based on Pseudoscience; Doesn't Kill Parasites or Cure Diseases - Science Feedback, 2024). This duality of hopeful testimonials and cautionary tales accentuates the divides within medical communities and public perception of alternative treatments (FTC v. Dr. Clark Research Association - Complaint, 2025).

Throughout this colorful mosaic of personal anecdotes, the narrative becomes clear: the zapper offers a purported alternative that some view as beneficial, despite its controversial standing. Stories of avoided surgeries and vanished ailments invigorate believers, inviting debate about placebo effects versus real efficacy. Charlotte's account of regained vitality post-zapper use exemplifies the spirit of Clark's proponents, who stand by their experiences as testimonies of change. Nevertheless, the lingering skepticism in the medical field remains, demanding a bridge between anecdotal evidence and stringent scientific validation (Hulda Clark's "Zapper" Device Is Based on Pseudoscience; Doesn't Kill Parasites or Cure Diseases - Science Feedback, 2024).

Balancing personal empowerment with medical prudence becomes paramount. While individual stories narrate intriguing successes, broader questions of safety and effectiveness persist. This mixed legacy of Hulda Clark's zapper exemplifies the complexities involved when embracing novel solutions in health care. The discussions stimulate deeper inquiries, challenging the boundaries of medical interventions while also celebrating personalized engagements with health and wellness journeys. Despite the current scientific consensus, the personal narratives surrounding the zapper ensure its continued discussion and interest as a polarizing element in health discourse.

## Concluding Thoughts

As the chapter wraps up, it's clear that Hulda Clark's zapper device represents more than an alternative treatment method; it marks a journey toward self-empowerment in health management. The stories of individuals like Charlotte, Alex, Maria, and many others—who continue to share positive feedback about Dr. Clark's protocols—highlight the powerful intersection of hope and personal empowerment in taking control of their own health.

Through their experiences, we see how stepping beyond conventional medical frameworks can yield profound outcomes, offering autonomy and reshaping narratives around healing. Looking ahead, these testimonies invite readers to explore further into the transformative potential of these methods, challenging traditional medical norms and embracing a future where personal choice plays a pivotal role in health care. As upcoming accounts delve into additional successes, such as children ceasing seizures and relief from chronic conditions, they will continue to illuminate new possibilities and inspire reevaluation of established health paradigms.

# Chapter 5: Standing Trial for Curing People

In the quiet border town of San Ysidro, California, Dr. Hulda Clark lived a modest life while carrying out the work that had made her both a beacon of hope and a target of controversy. Each day, she crossed the border into Tijuana, Mexico, where she operated a small clinic dedicated to what she believed was the most important mission of her life: helping people heal from diseases that modern medicine had failed to cure. Patients came from all over the world, drawn by her groundbreaking but unconventional protocols and the belief that the human body, when free of toxins and parasites, could heal itself—even from cancer.

But her quiet life and daily border crossings came to an abrupt end when she was arrested in San Diego and extradited back to Indiana to face charges of practicing medicine without a license—a case stemming from events nearly six years prior in Brown County. The arrest was a blow not just to Dr. Clark but to the countless supporters who saw her as a pioneer in alternative healing. Despite the legal threat and the possibility of two to eight years in prison, Clark remained undeterred.

"Ma'am, you are under arrest for practicing medicine without a license." The words echoed in the small California home, carrying the weight of confusion and disbelief. In that moment, amidst the clamor of police officers bustling around her, the elderly practitioner could hardly fathom how she had become the central figure in such a dramatic scene. Her life's work—helping people heal when conventional medicine had failed them—was being twisted into a criminal act. As she was led away in handcuffs, she wondered what had happened to the values of compassion and understanding that had always guided her path.

Across the country and beyond, this incident stirred a conversation much larger than one person's plight. It reflected a growing clash between innovation in healing practices and the strictures of traditional medical laws. This chapter delves into the intricate legal challenges faced by practitioners like her, shedding light on the broader implications of a system struggling to incorporate alternative methods. We will examine the societal and legal reverberations of daring to stand trial for curing people, exploring not only the individual battles but also the collective push towards greater medical freedom and choice.

# The Arrest and Legal Overreach

Indiana police arrived in California to arrest the 72-year-old practitioner for practicing unconventional medicine. This maneuver showcased a significant legal overreach, as officers crossed state lines to pursue someone whose only alleged crime was offering a type of care that defied the traditional norms. Her arrest signaled not just a targeting of her age but a broader message to those challenging the entrenched medical system. The image of her being apprehended in California for acts committed in Indiana emphasized a fundamental conflict between innovation in healthcare and the rigid boundaries of law that aim to uphold conventional standards. This movement was indicative of a legal system willing to stretch itself to its limits, invasively wedging between state sovereignties, to clamp down on what it perceived as burgeoning threats.

This isn't a typical case of law enforcement. Instead, it's an exemplar of enforcement taken to an extreme in the name of preserving a particular status quo. Here was a practitioner, whom many regarded as a healer, yet she was being dragged through a legal mudslide purely because her practices didn't conform. Her age alone should have warranted a degree of caution and humanity in enforcing the law, yet even that did not shield her from the cold reach of interstate enforcement. Her arrest was particularly poignant in revealing how far some authorities are willing to go to suppress practices they deem unorthodox. Here, crossing state boundaries became a metaphor for crossing ethical boundaries, highlighting an almost gladiatorial approach to maintaining control over medical practices.

As the Indiana authorities led her away, an echo of previous years when similar purges sought to quash dissent in various fields reverberated. These actions left no doubt about the seriousness with which traditional medical systems view non-compliance. They send a stern, unambiguous message to all practitioners who dare challenge conventional wisdom: step out of line, and expect forceful retribution. The legal complexities surrounding her arrest were manifold, but it fundamentally boiled down to protectionism in the guise of law enforcement. It was about more than just legal jurisdiction; it was about stamping authority over potential disruptors to the established order.

Such dramatic legal pursuits underscore the perceived threat she represented to orthodox medicine. It was as if her methods were somehow contagious, needing containment before they spread any further. Yet, the only virus at play was that of new thinking, something that apparently required immediate quarantine. By arresting her, a state was not just shackling an individual but attempting to cuff any ideas that might support her stance.

The encounter served as a preface to her ongoing battle, amplifying the daunting adversities she faced. It laid bare the enormous hurdles, both legal and emotional, as she danced with a justice system rigged to favor established medical entities. The arrest was a narrative device signaling there was no turning back—and that the stakes were life-altering. Its harshness fortified her resolve and added layers to the daunting challenge unfolding before her.

Despite these oppressive measures, the practitioner showed an extraordinary level of resilience. In an audacious display of commitment, she continued her work in Tijuana, crossing the border daily to offer care to American residents who could no longer avail themselves of her services stateside. Her determination illustrated a deep-seated devotion to her patients, transcending legal boundaries just as the Indiana police had crossed state lines.

Practicing in Tijuana marked a critical turning point in the story—an attempt to bypass the ipecac of legal quicksand applied by states wary of her rising influence. It demonstrated the tightrope she had to walk daily, balancing on the precipice of hope and defeat, armed only with her medical bag and unshakeable conviction. Her actions became a monologue of defiance in this David-and-Goliath narrative, cementing her place as a tenacious advocate for her angels.

Simply put, police action underscored the controversial space she occupied. While mainstream circles viewed her practices as infractions, others saw her as a bastion for patient rights and medical freedom. This dichotomy reflected how emotive and contentious the debate over conventional versus alternative medicine had become, with her plight casting a long shadow over future dialogues and policy decisions.

The silent roar of her defiance spoke volumes about her unwavering dedication to her patients. Despite the legal handcuffs, the metaphorical ones designed to curb her progressive approach, she ingeniously maneuvered within the constrained spaces left to her. She charted new courses, committing to small victories that flew under the radar. In Tijuana's clinic rooms, her expertise blossomed anew, navigating the careful seas between her country's backlash and the welcoming shores of medical outliers seeking help.

In the looming legal battles, this arrest's foundation became a pillar she leaned against, its rigidity amplifying her energy and determination to weather the burgeoning storm. As the narrative marches on, the foundational structure built with the story of her arrest offers a strong counterpoint to the systemic monolith she squares off against.

The stark severity of her arrest builds a poignant arc towards resilience and creativity—a thread weaving through the tapestry of law and medicine often overshadowed by politics. It crafts a robust connection to her ongoing tenacity and hints tantalizingly at the lengths to which the mind will go when duty calls. By standing trial for curing people, she becomes more than a practitioner; she is a spirit sowing seeds of her own mythos, one cross-border patient at a time.

## Practicing Against All Odds

Dr. Clark persisted despite the looming legal threats that had shadowed her for some time. Her determination was unyielding, and her decision to maintain her practice by relocating to Tijuana not only kept her work alive but also reflected her indomitable spirit and commitment to her patients. This move, however, set the stage for a significant legal battle that tested her resolve. Operating without formal recognition in a domain defined by regulation was a decision fraught with risk, yet she managed it with a blend of courage and tactical maneuvering.

"I'll be 71 next week," she told reporters, "and I'd like to spend the rest of my working days doing my research."

Her arrest only fueled international interest in her work. Messages of support poured in from around the globe—Sweden, Germany, South Africa, Japan, Australia, and across the United States—from people who credited her with saving their lives or giving them hope when conventional medicine had failed.

At the time of her arrest, Clark had just released her latest book, *The Cure for All Advanced Cancers*, a bold title that underscored her lifelong belief: that the causes and cures of disease were within reach, and that the public deserved to know the truth, no matter how fiercely the medical establishment tried to silence it.

Her trial commenced amidst a tense atmosphere filled with anticipation. Every detail of the proceedings mattered, as they would dictate her future and potentially shape the discourse around alternative healing practices. The courtroom became a theater of conflict between traditional law and the ideals of healing as a fundamental human right. Legal arguments centered around what constituted legitimate medical practice, examining whether an absence of formal licensure should invalidate her work or intentions.

Testimonies from her patients played a crucial role in the proceedings. These narratives brought human faces to what could have been a dry legal matter, shifting the focus to lived experiences rather than just abstract principles. Patients described how her care had improved their lives when conventional systems had failed them. A mother stood up to speak about her child's recovery, attributing it to Dr. Clark's unconventional yet effective methods. Her emphatic testimony brought raw emotion to the courtroom, creating ripples of empathy among the jurors.

Throughout this intense legal scrutiny, the defense team highlighted the ethical dimensions of her work. They argued that her practice was grounded in compassion and a deep commitment to health equity, challenging the notion that her lack of traditional credentials rendered her care ineffective or inherently dangerous. This argument resonated with jurors and the audience, raising questions about who gets to define what legitimate care constitutes and highlighting the arbitrarily narrow frameworks often employed to gatekeep the profession.

One key incident during the trial underscored the complexity of navigating these legal waters. A heated exchange occurred between the prosecution and the defense about the necessity and validity of formal training and credentials. The defense brought in expert witnesses who articulated that while formal education ensured a standard measure of competency, it wasn't the only route to effective medical practice. Their testimonies provided a robust counter-narrative to the prosecution's claims, framing Dr. Clark's work as a legitimate alternative approach. This discourse tapped into a wider debate about inclusivity and diversity within health services, illustrating that different paths could coexist within a broader healthcare ecosystem.

Adding another layer of complexity, the prosecution cited international border policies and the legal grey areas they created. This intersection of international law and healthcare highlighted how border dynamics complicated her work. Her decision to operate in Tijuana stemmed from practical necessity and pointed to broader systemic barriers hindering access to care. This was especially relevant in the context of restrictive US-Mexico border policies that exacerbated inequities in healthcare access (How Should Clinicians Express Solidarity with Asylum Seekers at the US-Mexico Border?, 2022).

Meanwhile, the defense painted her journey as one informed by the inability of traditional systems to accommodate the diverse needs of migrant populations. By setting up practice across the border, she circumvented certain barriers, echoing longstanding efforts to address such gaps in care on both micro and macro levels (Glass et al., 2022). This framing transformed her story from a solitary act of defiance into a broader commentary on the complexities of transnational healthcare provision.

Her eventual acquittal was met with a mix of relief and triumph, though it was not an unqualified victory. The verdict recognized the efficacy and indispensability of her care to her patients while quietly acknowledging that the established medical regulatory frameworks needed to evolve. The acquittal sent a broader message that shook conventional structures, suggesting that healing transcended borders and licenses.

This decision had implications that reached beyond her individual case. It hinted at a changing tide, one where innovation and necessity might push traditional systems to evolve or risk obsolescence. Her story was a beacon for those advocating for a more inclusive healthcare landscape that respected diversity in practice and approach.

As we move to explore the fallout from this verdict, it's clear that her acquittal wasn't just a personal win but a moment of possibility for alternative practices everywhere. It challenged entrenched systems, signaling that the future of healing might look different from its past. It heralded discussions that would amplify the tension between established medical norms and emerging practices that dared to push the boundaries, advocating for a system that embraced rather than excluded.

The upcoming sections will delve into the reverberations of her case, considering how the perception of unlicensed but effective practice affected broader medical systems. We will look at how this case fed into a narrative that framed alternative health practices not as sidelined outliers but as integral parts of an evolving healthcare system. Her story positions us at the cusp of a richer, more diverse dialogue about what it means to heal and to be healed in a world that constantly redefines itself.

# The Trial and Acquittal

Her journey to Tijuana spoke volumes of her commitment to patient care. Though banned in the United States, she crossed borders daily, displaying a resilience that seemed almost superhuman. This dedication rapidly became the catalyst for the events leading to her trial, painting her as a figurehead caught between her integrity and the rigid structures of medical legality.

The trial began, casting her in the role of a defendant facing charges of practicing medicine without a license. The courtroom bustled with expectant tension as the prosecution laid out its case, painting her as a rogue practitioner who circumvented regulations. Yet, the underlying narrative of her relentless commitment to serving those in need shone through the testimonies brought forward by her defense. Each witness from her patient roster spoke of their transformation under her care, their testimonials coloring the often sterile legal proceedings with vibrant hues of healing and gratitude. These stories narrated in court created a juxtaposition; they highlighted the divergence between established medical protocols and the simple efficacy of her practices.

Critical moments during the trial swayed opinions. A decisive point arrived when a patient, recovering from a debilitating condition after exhausting conventional treatments, shared an emotive testament. Through quivering sentences, they recounted how her unconventional methods provided relief and a semblance of normalcy. This narrative not only humanized her actions but also challenged the rigidity of the legal framework trying her. It encapsulated a sentiment echoed repeatedly—perhaps rules are not fit for those attempting to heal.

Her defense strategically leveraged such stories, crafting an argument around her methods' legitimacy rather than being an act of malpractice. Expert witnesses dissected the scientific reasoning behind her therapies, offering insights into how these could complement traditional approaches rather than undermine them. They positioned her as a pioneer for medical freedom, boldly walking where others would hesitantly tread, not out of defiance but genuine belief in the power of healing. This defense argument slowly chipped away at the prosecution's portrayal of her as a lawbreaker, shifting perception toward a more nuanced understanding of her role in this complex medical battle.

A pivotal scene in the courtroom involved an unexpected turn in legal interpretation. The judge, while summing up the case, suggested that the boundaries between legality and ethical duty to heal were not always clear-cut, thus feeding into the defense's narrative. This recognition seemed monumental. Her case was not just about legality but about questioning how far the law should extend in regulating the age-old art of healing. Such moments highlighted the reality of legal overreach, presenting it as a barrier rather than a protective measure.

The acquittal resonated beyond the courtroom. The decision not to convict echoed a wider understanding, suggesting that legal systems might sometimes lag behind the evolving landscapes of medical practices. Her vindication didn't just free her from legal bind—it was a watershed moment for alternative health practices, acknowledging their potential to coexist alongside mainstream medicine. This outcome reverberated as a siren call to regulatory bodies, emphasizing the need for laws that accommodate emerging healing practices rather than stifle them.

This trial, beyond personal victory, symbolized a pivot toward inclusivity in medicine. Her story mirrored those of many unsung practitioners whose work, though often ostracized, held the promise of relief where conventional medicine fell short. By choosing not to convict, the judiciary inadvertently endorsed a rethinking of medical jurisdiction where the act of curing became less about following set paths and more about meeting the patients' needs where they stood.

As the section concludes, her acquittal is less viewed as a personal gain and more as a systemic challenge. It sends ripples across the alternative health community, emboldening practitioners to pursue their art with renewed vigor. Conversely, it throws open a gauntlet to regulatory bodies, urging them to recalibrate and consider if their policies genuinely serve the evolving needs of doctor and patient alike (Criminal Convictions and Medical Licensure, 2011).

This verdict will not easily be forgotten, nestled at the forefront of debates on medical freedom versus regulatory jurisdiction. It frames the conversation on whether healing should be confined by borders, metaphorically and legally. In this light, the act of curing without a license becomes a subversive act aimed at toppling systemic barriers; the reverse side of the coin is a rallying cry for patient-first practices, unshackled by rigid conformities (Medical News., 1903).

As this tale perpetuates and unfolds, the journey from legal acquittal to broader change awaits. The ramifications of her case mark a significant bend in the road, exploring deeper implications in the chapter that follows, while her story remains a cornerstone of an ongoing dialogue.

## Implications of Curing without a License

In the aftermath of Dr. Clark's dramatic acquittal, we witness a daring pushback against the rigid systems governing medical practice. This individual's journey disrupts not only the lives saved by her unconventional methods but also the creaky edifice of officialdom in medical regulation. Why does curing people without a sanctioned license pose such a threat? The answer lies at the heart of a struggle as old as medicine itself, a battle balancing the preservation of human health with financial interests and regulatory controls.

Venture into how alternative practices like those of our protagonist challenge the status quo. When a practitioner employs a method outside sanctioned boundaries, it forces us to scrutinize not only the treatments used but also the regulatory frameworks that impose such limits. Many health practitioners argue that these controls exist for valid reasons—ensuring safety, efficacy, and fairness in treatments offered to the public. However, is it possible they also maintain a balance of power leaning heavily in favor of traditional medical pathways and pharmaceutical interest? Governments, with vested interests in controlling public health, react decisively when their territory encroaches on unapproved methods. The licensing systems crafted to safeguard public health can sometimes struggle to integrate innovative treatments quickly, resulting in tension between innovation and regulation (Wong, 2020).

Take the global issue of compulsory licensing during health emergencies as an example. Chile and Ecuador set up legal frameworks for issuing compulsory licenses, ensuring their populations receive necessary COVID-19 treatments without succumbing to monopolistic pricing (Wong, 2020). In contrast, alternative treatments for other diseases remain entangled in bureaucratic procedures. If a similar approach were more broadly adopted, as seen during other medical crises, perhaps alternative treatments wouldn't incite fear of instability but rather an evolution in medical care (Wong, 2020).

The public embodies another layer of complexity. The perception of medical legitimacy relies heavily on public trust in licensed professionals. Patients often view sanctioned treatments as safe, trusting healthcare systems to protect them from unproven practices. However, growing discontent with certain conventional treatments prompts some patients to seek alternatives, especially when traditional options prove ineffective or costly. This shift subtly undermines the authority of established medical regulations, painting alternative practitioners as custodians of knowledge beyond government's therapeutic approval. How can traditional practitioners and regulatory bodies ensure public safety without stifling innovative alternatives?

Consider, for instance, how countries bound by free-trade agreements might fear trade retaliations when using compulsory licenses for medications. This mirrors the hesitancy regulators face worldwide when confronting unlicensed cures threatening established economic interests (Wong, 2020). In a free market, introducing less costly and potentially more effective treatment introduces a formidable competitor for entrenched pharmaceutical juggernauts. Financial interests inevitably weave into the fabric of health policy, shaping the environments where alternative methods fight for legitimacy.

Case studies from the past, like the HIV/AIDS epidemic, show government cooperation with organizations like Médecins Sans Frontières necessary to deploy affordable solutions (Wong, 2020). Those advocating for alternative medicine need similar partnerships to reduce suspicion, promoting understanding between traditional and novel approaches. Establishing alliances, cooperative platforms, and knowledge exchanges strengthens alternative practitioners' legal and social positions within the medical community (Wong, 2020).

As compelling as these measures might be, they should avoid redundancy and touch on how individual cases, like our protagonist's acquittal, come to symbolize greater phenomena. Her victory stirs conversations around medical autonomy and patient choice, driving home the argument that healing shouldn't rest solely in the hands of historically dominant entities. This applies especially to practitioners skilled in holistic, non-traditional therapies, often fighting an uphill battle to rescue their reputations and practices from legal condemnation.

It's worth illustrating the subtle psychological warfare waged in courtrooms and public opinion arenas. Practitioners face fiery opposition, cast as charlatans on one hand or rebels breaking chains of outdated systems on the other. By challenging the idea that healing lives in a regulated box, this trial and its outcome mark the opening of a Pandora's box for traditional practitioners striving to keep alternative methods under their purview. This shift in perception might soften hardline stances against experimental treatments that can, under scrutiny and transparency, serve various populations and health crises.

Regulators' inertia often means patients wait unnecessarily for life-altering innovations to clear arduous approval processes, placing alternative medicine in a unique position to fill that gap swiftly yet safely (Wong, 2020). Historical reticence from both medical and regulatory institutions in integrating these options means alternative health practices often seep into the system informally at first. If mainstream healthcare incorporated qualified alternative practitioners sooner, the tension between structured regulation and free-form healing might lessen.

Delve into how shifts in healthcare regulation can illuminate pathways for practitioners trailblazing new treatment avenues. As we've seen from initiatives tackling COVID-19 (Wong, 2020), a framework for swift governmental response in approving new methods is necessary. Regulatory bodies need nimble protocols to evaluate and integrate proven alternative methods. Coupled with strict conditions and a watchful public eye, such mechanisms would ensure safety while nurturing innovation.

This revolutionary landscape may proffer not just the single practitioner a second chance, but a broader movement a platform solidified through shared trials, victories won in courtrooms, and ongoing dialogue with health authorities. Together, these pieces form an evolving mosaic depicting a healthcare future where healing doesn't demand bureaucracy but champions universal accessibility and scientific excellence.

# Final Analysis

Dr. Clark's journey highlights the enduring tension between innovation and regulation within the healthcare landscape, casting her as a pivotal figure in the quest for medical freedom. Her acquittal is not just a win for her but a triumph for alternative health seekers everywhere who dare to question mainstream medical practices. With courageous defiance, she challenged the conventional boundaries, and her story inspires countless others facing similar trials. The verdict echoes a call for compassion over regulations, hinting at a future where healing transcends traditional confines, encouraging us to rethink how we define legitimate care. As her tale underscores the potential of alternative approaches, it opens the door to dialogues about inclusivity, patient choice, and the realignment of regulatory frameworks with evolving healthcare needs. Now more than ever, this narrative invites us to envision a world where diverse healing methods coexist, championing an inclusive system that acknowledges and integrates innovative paths to wellness. By embracing such possibilities, we can foster a healthcare environment that celebrates varied routes to healing, offering hope and empowerment to those left unheard by conventional medicine.

# Chapter 6 The Global Movement She Sparked

Dr. Alan Baklayan remembers the day he first encountered Dr. Hulda Clark's theories—a moment that transformed his career and would eventually ripple across Europe. As a passionate naturopath in Germany, Baklayan had been seeking innovative ways to address chronic health issues plaguing his patients. Despite being intrigued by Clark's unconventional approach, many of his peers met her ideas with skepticism. Yet, Baklayan couldn't shake the feeling that there was something more to her protocols than dismissed claims or anecdotal evidence.

This sense of urgency led him to delve deeper, testing these methods within his practice. Soon, stories began emerging from his patients—people reporting improvements where conventional treatments had failed them. These were not just isolated incidents but a growing body of testimonials suggesting real potential in Clark's methods. While some remained doubtful, Baklayan witnessed firsthand the impact these protocols could have, which set the stage for a wider acceptance across Europe. His journey exemplified a broader narrative: when faced with unyielding medical challenges, people are willing to explore beyond traditional medicine. This chapter explores how Clark's influence spread internationally, reshaping perceptions and practices far beyond its origins.

## Dr. Alan Baklayan's contributions

Dr. Alan Baklayan's contributions have played a crucial role in validating and advancing Dr. Hulda Clark's parasite-fungus theory within Europe, particularly in Germany. A key figure in naturopathic medicine, Baklayan has applied Clark's methods in innovative ways, helping to solidify her protocols' reputation and adoption in the alternative health community. His work is significant because it provides a scientific basis for Clark's theories, which some had regarded with skepticism. By focusing on research and practical applications, Baklayan has helped shift perceptions of Clark's ideas, promoting them as viable treatment options for a range of health issues.

Baklayan's practice in Germany integrates various tests for detecting parasites and fungi, echoing Clark's approach. By personalizing treatments using Clark's zapper device and specific herbal remedies, he empowers patients with chronic health problems to achieve better outcomes. This aligns with Clark's principle that many health issues originate from parasitic and fungal infections, which can be mitigated through targeted protocols. The successful application of these treatments in Germany fosters broader acceptance, and Baklayan's pioneering efforts are regularly cited in realms of alternative medicine for their effectiveness.

The adoption of these methods is not limited to Germany. They have found a firm foothold in nearby countries, such as Switzerland and Italy. In Switzerland, practitioners incorporate Clark's protocols in mainstream alternative health clinics, where patients often report improved health and resilience. These clinics emphasize holistic care, a concept central to Clark's ideology, which considers the whole person rather than isolated symptoms. Swiss practitioners also express appreciation for the comprehensive nature of Clark's methods, extending their reach and credibility across health care systems.

In Italy, Clark's protocols continue to thrive within various clinics. The Italian medical community's openness towards integrative medicine provides fertile ground for the principles set forth by Clark, spearheaded by practitioners inspired by Baklayan's success in Germany. Italian clinics host workshops and training sessions for health professionals, introducing Clark's methods and demonstrating their potential in patient care. Such educational initiatives further legitimize and disseminate her practices, allowing more health care providers to understand and utilize these innovative treatment options.

The impact of adopting Clark's theories stretches across the entire European alternative health scene. Since Clark's protocols emphasize prevention and patient empowerment, they resonate well with individuals seeking proactive health management over conventional treatments. This trend is evident in testimonials and case studies from patients who have experienced significant improvement, often detailing how Clark's methods served as the turning point in managing their chronic conditions. The real-life successes of Baklayan's patients play a central role in substantiating the efficacy of these protocols in health circles.

Renowned figures in the health community, particularly those in alternative medicine, also leverage Clark's theories. Professionals in holistic and integrative practices often highlight Baklayan's work as a model for merging traditional principles with modern approaches to treatment. The fusion aligns with increasing global interest in personalized medicine, which relies on understanding individual differences for effective care—Clark's protocols fit neatly within this progressive wave.

The broader implication of Clark's acceptance in Europe is the growing curiosity and respect for alternative health methodologies. The integration of Clark's theories prompts regulatory and research bodies to explore these approaches more seriously, leading to dialogues around their potential integration into more conventional medical frameworks. As awareness increases, European clinics become hotspots for patients worldwide seeking alternatives to conventional treatments. The movement enables a thriving exchange of information and best practices among international practitioners.

In summary, Dr. Alan Baklayan's validation of Clark's parasite-fungus theory in Germany has paved the way for broader acceptance across Europe, particularly in Switzerland and Italy. Clinics in these regions have successfully implemented Clark's methods, demonstrating their value and enhancing their legitimacy within the alternative health sector. Concrete outcomes and testimonials exemplify the effectiveness of these protocols, driving interest and adoption in mainstream medical communities. This evolution signifies a pivotal shift within European health care, emphasizing the importance of holistic and personalized treatment in improving patient outcomes.

Looking forward, the continent's embrace of Clark's methods sets a foundation for further exploration and integration. Clinics continue to share insights and improvements drawn from Clark's theories, suggesting a persistent and expanding influence on international alternative health practices. This paves the way for a future where harmonizing traditional and modern health methodologies offers a comprehensive resource for global wellness.

As the narrative progresses, we delve into the work of Dr. Adolfo Panfili in Italy. Known for his role as a physician to Pope John Paul II, Dr. Panfili's incorporation of Clark's protocols highlights another dimension of European acceptance, illustrating their wide-ranging appeal and adaptability. This underscores the diverse applications and potential of these methodologies, reinforcing their relevance and potential impact in the broader context of global health developments.

# A Vatican Doctor's Support

When you think of the international shift towards alternative medicine, it's impossible not to mention the profound influence of Dr. Hulda Clark's theories. Dr. Alan Baklayan, who validated Clark's parasite-fungus theory, played a crucial role in introducing her methodologies to clinics across Germany, Switzerland, and Italy. This paved the way for the broader acceptance of her protocols. Enter Dr. Adolfo Panfili, whose implementation of Clark's methods in Italy signifies an era of growing validation and adoption. Recognized as the physician to Pope John Paul II, Panfili's use of Clark's protocols marks a significant shift towards integrating alternative therapies within mainstream healthcare.

Dr. Panfili, an advocate of integrative medicine, combined conventional medical practices with alternative therapies. His educational background, deeply rooted in conventional medicine, provided him with a firm foundation. Yet, it was his openness to exploring new methods that led to the adoption of Clark's protocols. By using these in his practice, Panfili showcased the effectiveness of methods that were often met with skepticism by the traditional medical community. His endorsement came not only from his medical expertise but also from his reputed association with the Vatican. Imagine the credibility this lent to Clark's methods. In a country where the Catholic Church holds significant sway, Panfili's influence was substantial.

Specific examples from Panfili's practice highlight the effectiveness of Clark's methods. Consider the case of a patient suffering from chronic fatigue, a condition often labeled elusive by traditional medicine. With a regimen that included Clark's parasite cleanses, the patient reported significant improvements. These cases are more than anecdotal; they serve as testimonials to the methodologies Panfili employed. The narratives coming from his patients further fueled interest in Clark's therapies. When people experience tangible improvements, it's hard to argue with results.

Dr. Panfili's professional journey illustrates how he integrates various aspects of medical science with innovative alternatives. His holistic approach, which includes not only Clark's protocols but also other complementary remedies, reflects a nuanced understanding of health. This method considers the entire being rather than a single symptom or condition. It's a shift that resonates with many seeking health solutions outside conventional parameters. Panfili's success stories not only extended Clark's influence but also bridged a critical gap between traditional and alternative medicine in Italy.

Beyond the walls of his clinic, Panfili's endorsement carried weight across Europe, inspiring confidence in Clark's systems among healthcare providers and the public. His work demonstrated that alternative treatments could coalesce with conventional practices to produce better health outcomes. The Pope's physician endorsing such methods was no small matter. It sparked a conversation about the potential benefits of integrating alternative therapies into mainstream healthcare. In Italy, this conversation resonated with a burgeoning movement towards embracing holistic and complementary treatments.

As practitioners and the public increasingly explored these methodologies, Clark's influence spread further. By establishing a network of practitioners interested in alternative medicine, Panfili contributed to a widening acceptance of Clark's approaches. His work created ripple effects not only in Italy but also in nearby regions. Practitioners began incorporating Clark's protocols into their own practices, sometimes developing innovative variations that suited local needs and health cultures.

The momentum generated by advocates like Dr. Panfili laid a foundation for organized initiatives that sought to further research and organize Clark's methods systematically. This leads us to the formation of the Dr. Clark Research Association, founded by David Amrein. This organization didn't arise in a vacuum. It was the logical extension of the ground broken by Panfili and others. The association aimed to compile evidence, share insights, and support practitioners who used Clark's methods. This network became a hub for exchanging ideas, learning from one another, and collectively advancing alternative medicine research.

The creation of the Dr. Clark Research Association marked a significant step toward institutionalizing and thereby legitimizing the practices that many had embraced anecdotally. Organized efforts allowed for structured research and validation, which served to expand the reach of Clark's theories beyond isolated practitioners to a more organized community focused on alternative therapies. This represents a crucial shift from individual practice to community engagement, influencing broader public perceptions and acceptance.

By connecting practitioners globally, Amrein's organization brought scientific rigor to the table, conducting studies that sought to verify the claims made about Clark's protocols. With results published and shared widely, this enabled more practitioners to consider and adopt these methods. Panfili's initial endorsement provided the credibility needed to pique interest, but the association provided the empirical backing that further solidified Clark's place within the broader health discourse.

In essence, practitioners like Dr. Panfili shine a light on the transformative potential of blending alternative and traditional medicine. The validation and global movement sparked by their work have opened doors for countless individuals seeking comprehensive health solutions. Whether it's through the endorsement of a respected physician or an organized research group, the impact on healthcare paradigms underscores a pivotal moment in medicine's evolution. It challenges the status quo and invites a future where health is viewed holistically, with openness to therapies that go beyond conventional boundaries.

## Clark's Methods Sweep Across Europe

Building on the momentum established by Dr. Adolfo Panfili in Italy, Dr. Hulda Clark's health protocols began sweeping across Europe, creating a transformative movement. Dr. Panfili's application of Clark's methods drew attention to their potential, prompting health seekers across various countries to explore these alternative options. As Clark's theories migrated beyond the borders of Italy, they gained traction by tapping into a growing demand for holistic and non-conventional treatments, leading to significant influence and application across Europe and beyond.

Clark's protocols, particularly parasite cleanses, liver detoxes, and Zapper devices, quickly became subjects of interest. Each of these methods offered unique solutions to health issues that conventional medicine often struggles to address. Parasite cleanses, for instance, focus on eliminating harmful organisms from the body. With the claim of improving digestive health, increasing energy levels, and addressing a range of chronic conditions, they attracted those skeptical of traditional treatments. Liver detoxes operate under the premise of clearing toxins accumulated from modern lifestyles, promising benefits like enhanced liver function and clearer skin, which resonated with individuals conscious of their body's detoxification processes. Zapper devices, small electrical units designed to kill parasites, viruses, and bacteria via electrical frequencies, complemented these cleanses by providing an at-home, technology-driven approach to health intervention.

The popularity of these protocols soared as word spread around alternative health circles. Dr. Clark's work was frequently featured at international health expos, where practitioners demonstrated these methods to eager audiences. One of the major highlights was the annual Mind, Body, Spirit festival in London, where hundreds gathered to learn about and experience these alternative therapies firsthand. Practitioners and health advocates displayed how these methods aligned with the ever-growing drive towards self-empowerment in health. Testimonials and case studies presented at these expos often revealed stories of chronic illness sufferers experiencing newfound relief, many attributing their improved health to regular parasite cleanses and the strategic use of Zapper devices.

In Germany, for example, several natural health clinics have incorporated Clark's methods into their offerings, driven by consumer interest in non-pharmaceutical solutions. These clinics reported an increase in bookings for consultations and therapies related to liver detoxes and parasite management, often emphasizing a holistic approach that integrates diet alterations and lifestyle changes alongside Clark's protocols. France saw the emergence of local groups dedicated to Clark's methods, hosting workshops and meetings where they shared experiences and advice on using these protocols effectively.

Practitioners like Dr. Klaus Faber in Austria went so far as to establish centers entirely dedicated to Clark's teachings, offering a range of services from educational seminars to hands-on treatment sessions. Dr. Faber often cites a client, Renate, whose struggles with autoimmune diseases saw remarkable improvement following a regiment of liver detoxes and the use of Zapper technology. Renate's story mirrors those of many who turned to these methods in search of options beyond what traditional medicine offers. Such narratives, spread through word of mouth and online platforms, created an expanding network of believers and participants.

Dr. Clark's methods resonated strongly with Alternative Health Seekers, who valued non-invasive, natural prevention strategies, and Medical Freedom Advocates, who pushed for the right to choose their medical pathways free from state-imposed mandates. Chronic Illness Sufferers, in search of hope and relief after exhausting mainstream options, found solace in Clark's theories which often delivered results unattainable through conventional means. Moreover, Truth Seekers, skeptical of mainstream narratives, embraced Clark's approaches as part of a broader quest for authentic, uncharted solutions to health problems they perceived as inadequately addressed by conventional systems.

A compelling metaphor often shared among these community members describes Clark's protocols as a key to unlocking a fogged-up window. They don't claim to change the scenery but clear up the view, allowing the individual's natural health to drive their well-being. This metaphor underscores the idea that the individual, with the right tools, can reclaim control over their health journey.

As the movement continued to prosper, the next wave of expansion saw these methods reach entirely new audiences outside Europe. Clinics in Australia and South Africa reported increasing interest in Clark's protocols, driven by similar motivations and desires for alternative health solutions. The spread of parasite cleanses, liver detoxes, and Zapper devices continued to find fertile ground among global audiences, eagerly taking up the cause.

The widespread adoption and continued proliferation of these practices led to international discourse about the efficacy and ethical implications of such alternative therapies. This discussion highlights the balance between conventional medical advice and the rights of individuals to pursue non-traditional treatments. Moving forward, this debate will play a crucial role as the next section explores how the increasing adoption of these methods has prompted reactions and adaptations from diverse audiences around the world.

# Booming Support in Europe of Clark's Methods

The awareness spread by David Amrein through the Dr. Clark Research Association opened significant channels for the acceptance of Hulda Clark's protocols. This moves beyond mere awareness; it lays the groundwork for practical application in various parts of the world, especially in Europe where her methods have found fertile ground. With increasing popularity, these practices create a ripple effect influencing both individuals and communities about alternative health options.

In Europe, there's a notable shift toward embracing natural health remedies, and Clark's protocols, such as parasite cleanses, liver detoxes, and Zapper devices, are at the forefront of this movement. The core attraction of these methods lies in their promise to address health issues holistically, without the side effects commonly associated with conventional medicine. The public, increasingly skeptical of pharmaceuticals that often come with a lengthy list of possible adverse reactions, is turning to solutions that emphasize well-being and preventive care.

Take, for example, the city of Berlin, known for its pioneering ventures in health and wellness. Here, the adoption of Clark's methodologies has made its way into small wellness clinics and larger health centers alike. These establishments promote parasite cleanses as a way to improve digestive health and boost energy levels. People relate to the idea of cleansing the body from within, seeing it as a proactive approach to staving off illness.

London, long a hub for alternative therapies, has witnessed a similar embrace. The popularity of liver detoxing regimens that stem from Clark's recommendations reflects the broader acceptance of detoxification in the UK. This method's appeal is its simplicity and perceived effectiveness, offering a feeling of rejuvenation and resetting of the body's natural balance. Reports of increased vitality and better general health after these detoxes circulate widely, encouraging more to explore these natural avenues.

Zapper devices, initially met with skepticism, have grown in popularity due to their claimed effectiveness in addressing various ailments without medical intervention. The concept of electrically stimulating the body to eliminate pathogens aligns with a tech-savvy Europe that is increasingly interested in innovative health gadgets. Community workshops and health seminars regularly feature demonstrations of these devices, fostering a hands-on understanding of their use and benefits. Evaluation and advocacy by holistic practitioners lend credibility, further integrating these devices into everyday health practices.

Across the continent, the growing popularity of Clark's methods echoes a broader trend: a return to nature and simpler, non-invasive health solutions that connect deeply with personal health beliefs. There's also an educational component; people are not just following these protocols blindly but are engaging with and understanding the principles behind them. This informed participation boosts the credibility and sustainability of Clark's global movement.

In Scandinavian countries, the connection to nature has always been a part of cultural identity, so the integration of natural health practices isn't unexpected. Clark's protocols fit seamlessly into the societal fabric that values organic and holistic lifestyles. Nordic citizens, often seen participating in outdoor activities and mindful of nature's cycles, see great compatibility with parasite cleanses and liver detoxification rituals that synchronize with particular times of the year when daylight varies drastically.

Similarly, in countries like France and Spain, where tradition and modernity blend beautifully, the appeal of Clark's protocols lies in their embrace of natural remedies that have been part of the cultural heritage. Franco Spanish interest in herbs and natural solutions complements these cleansing protocols, which are easily adapted into family traditions and wellness routines.

The global spread of Clark's influence isn't just geographical but also deeply social. Social media and community exchange play a pivotal role in this expansion. Platforms dedicated to natural health are spaces where users share experiences, tips, and successes with Clark's methods, creating online communities of like-minded individuals. These forums act as sources of information and support, propelling the movement forward.

However, it's crucial to examine why these protocols continue to resonate with people today. One reason is the disenchantment with conventional healthcare systems that seem impersonal and often inaccessible. Private clinics and personalized wellness plans, focusing on Clark's methods, offer a counterbalance to this bureaucratic approach, emphasizing personal agency and individualized care.

Moreover, the philosophy behind Clark's approach dovetails seamlessly with an eco-friendly ethos, valuing sustainability and respect for natural resources. This synergy with modern environmental consciousness makes adopting such lifestyles attractive and socially responsible, supporting a healthier planet and society.

Also, as chronic conditions increasingly burden healthcare systems, individuals seek preventative measures to maintain health rather than reacting to symptoms. These methods provide an alternative approach that encourages regular maintenance of health rather than crisis management, aligning with an evolving understanding of wellness that is proactive rather than reactive.

These cultural shifts hint at a more profound transformation as understanding grows and acceptance spreads globally. People are carving their paths toward well-being, supported by Clark's legacy of health empowerment. Europe and other regions embracing these methods move closer toward holistic health experiences rooted in connecting body, mind, and lifestyle choices in a cohesive journey toward overall wellness.

The global movement sparked by Clark continues to thrive, building on the foundations of her holistic vision, encouraging people worldwide to look within and beyond the conventional. This not only redefines health approaches but also reshapes societal views on what it means to live healthily in the 21st century. Her influence is immortalized in every choice made toward natural healing, a testament to her impact on many lives globally.

Insights and Implications

In this chapter, we've journeyed through the remarkable spread of Dr. Hulda Clark's theories across Europe, driven by pioneers like Dr. Alan Baklayan and Dr. Adolfo Panfili. Their advocacy and application of Clark's parasite-fungus theory have transformed skepticism into acceptance, positioning these protocols as credible options in alternative medicine circles from Germany to Italy. The integration of Clark's methods in various European clinics underscores a grassroots shift towards natural and personalized health solutions, resonating with those disenchanted by conventional treatments. Crucially, this movement is not just about alternative health practices but about empowering individuals with tools for self-directed healing—a notion that aligns with broader desires for autonomy in health choices. Now, as Clark's influence continues to grow, practitioners and patients are poised to explore even greater synergies between traditional and modern approaches, fostering a global dialogue on holistic health that emphasizes prevention, empowerment, and the healing potential within us all.

# Chapter 7 If She Was Wrong, Why Were People Getting Healed?

Picture a woman named Lisa standing at the crossroads of hope and despair. For years, she suffered from relentless chronic pain that mainstream medicine couldn't seem to alleviate. Desperate for relief, she quietly turned away from her daily regimen of prescribed medications and sought solace in the whispers of alternative therapies: acupuncture, herbal remedies, and meditation. Skeptics around her scoffed, questioning the legitimacy of these "unproven" methods. Yet, to Lisa's astonishment, not only did her pain subside, but she found herself revitalized, living proof of the healing potential that lay beyond conventional borders.

Lisa's journey isn't unique. Many like her have turned to alternative treatments, seeking answers where traditional paths failed them. This chapter delves into why mainstream medicine often dismisses these alternatives, what role financial interests play in this dynamic, and whether the criticisms leveled against unconventional approaches truly hold weight. Through exploring these questions, we'll uncover deeper insights into the intricate web linking medical practices, patient outcomes, and the ever-persistent quest for genuine healing.

# Avoidance by Mainstream Medicine

Alternative treatments often sit at the periphery of mainstream medical acceptance, despite persistent anecdotal success stories. People turn to holistic and natural cures when conventional options fail them, yet mainstream establishments often choose to dismiss these alternatives out of ignorance or skepticism. But why?

One compelling reason is the deeply entrenched influence of pharmaceutical companies in medical research and practice. These companies invest substantial resources in traditional medicine development. As a result, the financial interests tied to pharmaceuticals create intense pressure on medical institutions and practitioners to adhere strictly to standardized treatment methods, often disregarding lesser-known therapies that lack big-budget research backing. For instance, patients have frequently attested to the benefits of alternative practices like acupuncture or herbal supplements when tackling chronic pain or autoimmune diseases. Yet, these methods tend to be sidelined because they don't align with conventional priorities or profit models.

Critics argue that because alternative treatments don't always undergo the rigors of double-blind clinical trials, their value gets brushed off. But is it really the lack of clinical validation that sees alternative methods discredited, or is it a reluctance to explore outside the parameters set by pharmaceutical-driven research agendas? The latter argument has some merit when considering that historical trends show mainstream medicine's aversion to therapies not backed by significant research. This skepticism pertains not only to patient safety but also to the perceived threat to the conventional medical establishment's authority and credibility.

Consider the case of treatments for chronic illnesses such as fibromyalgia or chronic fatigue syndrome. Patients have reported finding relief through methods like diet modifications, yoga, or certain supplements—approaches often dismissed by skeptics due to the lack of government grants or corporate funding supporting such methods. The mainstream's tendency to disregard these is not just about doubt over efficacy; it's about maintaining the power dynamics and financial coherence of medicine that rests heavily on pharmaceutical funding.

This skepticism has roots in broader socio-cultural narratives, as documented in research highlighting overarching gender biases in medical treatment and diagnosis. For instance, women have historically been underrepresented in clinical trials and, consequently, their unique health needs are often ignored by mainstream medicine, as observed by the lack of research into diseases affecting female reproductive health (Admin, 2021). Similarly, alternative medicine often caters to those who feel marginalized by the existing healthcare framework, drawing interest from demographics traditionally neglected or mismanaged by mainstream practitioners, like women or those with chronic conditions.

Openness to non-traditional healing methods doesn't just resonate with dissatisfaction stemming from specific health disparities but also reflects an increasing distrust of a healthcare system that seems more loyal to pharmaceutical profits than patient outcomes. The medical field's wariness towards alternative treatments has its roots in this dance between profit and patient care (Patricia Edmonds, 2019). The pharmaceutical industry's grip not only prioritizes patented drugs over easily accessible remedies but also influences medical education, steering graduates towards algorithmic treatment protocols rather than holistic patient care approaches.

Many proponents of alternative medicine argue for a system that looks beyond clinical settings for healing methods that align more closely with natural physiological rhythms and mental wellness. In doing so, they not only oppose the ethics of pharmaceutical influence but also advocate for more patient-centric and culturally adaptive healthcare practices. There's a pressing need for formal acknowledgment of therapies that align with diverse lived experiences and cultural backgrounds and not merely Western-centric medical tenets.

Social interest in alternative techniques also stems from a deeper philosophical stance on personal autonomy and bodily integrity in relation to health services. People turning to alternative therapies often express a desire to regain control over their health journey, free from pharmaceutical side-effect profiles or indifferent clinical settings. This desire for autonomy clearly intersects with broader debates on medical freedoms and personal liberties, echoing socio-political sentiments advocating personal choice over corporate-influenced mandates.

Despite a modernized front, traditional medicine remains deeply conservative, often firmly wedded to established norms and singularly focused on evidence-based approaches that, while valid, aren't always exhaustive in capturing the full spectrum of health and wellness possibilities. This can create an antagonistic environment where alternative methods are mocked rather than considered for their potential contributions. Integrating alternative practices more openly can address these gaps, aligning medicine better with the varied ways individuals experience and interpret their health needs.

While mainstream medicine offers remarkable advancements in treating acute illnesses and life-threatening conditions, its limitations become apparent with chronic, subjective, or non-uniform health challenges. These are the arenas where alternative medicine thrives, not as replacements, but as complements offering additional insights into humanity's complex relationship with health.

Solutions may lie in greater recognition of a collaborative healthcare model, where traditional and alternative practices coalesce, leading to enriched, patient-centered care. By harnessing the strengths of both, society can work towards a more holistic view of healing. Mainstream institutions must recognize the value of exploring alternative avenues not merely as a necessity for some, but as a means to enrich the overall tapestry of healthcare knowledge. As interest in alternative methods grows alongside a call for personal autonomy, the medical establishment must reassess its resistance, reconciling financial incentives with the ethical imperative to prioritize patient-centered, diverse, and inclusive healthcare solutions.

## Traditional Criticisms Analyzed

Mainstream medicine often dismisses alternative practitioners, mocking them instead of seriously considering their potential. This behavior sets a foundation for understanding the scientific gatekeeping mechanisms primarily controlled by pharmaceutical interests. In a landscape where financial influences heavily dictate treatment credibility, alternative therapies frequently find themselves sidelined. The question isn't just about scientific validation but about who holds sway over the purse strings funding the research and clinical trials determining a treatment's acceptance.

Scientific gatekeeping operates like a highly selective club, where pharmaceutical funding dictates the guest list. The process tends to favor treatments that promise substantial returns on investment, aligning with the business models of big pharma companies rather than prioritizing holistic health outcomes. This selective financial backing often steers research directions, ensuring that costly and lucrative pharmaceuticals get priority over potentially groundbreaking but less profitable alternatives. Such dynamics create challenges for alternative medicine, confining it to the fringes and often branding it as non-scientific. In this scenario, lack of peer review and clinical trials isn't necessarily a reflection of ineffectiveness but rather a consequence of being sidelined by more influential financial stakeholders.

The dismissal of alternatives doesn't necessarily stem from scientific inadequacy but rather from the structure of incentivization. Consider the example of Dr. Johanna Budwig, a German biochemist who developed a dietary protocol claimed to aid in cancer treatment. Despite anecdotal success stories, she faced harsh criticism and dismissal from the medical establishment, largely due to the absence of formal clinical trials and peer-reviewed studies. This sidelining persisted even as many patients reported better health outcomes. However, without the substantial backing or vested interest from major pharmaceutical companies, her work remained outside the mainstream conversation. Her case underscores a larger pattern where financial interests, rather than pure scientific inquiry, guide the dialogue on treatment efficacy.

Take also the controversial story of laetrile, a compound derived from apricot pits, once heralded as a potential cancer treatment. Although widely used in alternative circles and backed by testimonies of its efficacy, laetrile was never embraced by mainstream medicine. Official studies declared it ineffective, yet these findings quickly sparked debate over whether the studies had genuine scientific intent or if they served to reinforce pharmaceutical interests. The gatekeeping here arguably wasn't just about protecting patients from ineffective treatments, but of safeguarding the financial ecosystems surrounding conventional oncology, supported by multi-million-dollar investments in chemotherapy drugs and radiation technology.

The influence of pharmaceutical funding is further apparent in research prioritization. Access to financial support can determine which hypotheses graduate from theory to tested practice. Pharmaceutical companies, driven by patent profit incentives, typically choose to invest in treatments that can be patented and monetized rather than natural substances that don't offer the same financial leverage. This choice inevitably limits the scope of scientific exploration and assessment of genuinely promising alternatives.

The lack of peer-reviewed publications for many alternative treatments doesn't necessarily reflect their scientific unviability. Rather, it underscores the difficulties faced in obtaining the necessary funding and institutional backing to embark on the rigorous and costly peer review process. The structure currently in place raises questions about missed opportunities and stifled innovations. The pathway from anecdotal evidence to scientifically accepted treatment is full of hurdles that many financially unsupported therapies cannot surmount.

Discussing these biases leads to a broader critique of the peer review system itself. While theoretically a hallmark of scientific integrity, it can become an instrument of exclusion when coupled with financial biases. Given the potential for bias or manipulation within peer review—ranging from reviewers who harbor conflicts of interest to journals prioritizing research aligned with funding sources—such influences can directly impact which findings gain traction. As Systematic Review articulates, "the practice of peer review is based on faith in its effects, rather than on facts" (Smith, 2006). This faith might unwittingly preserve a status quo that favors more profitable medicinal endeavors.

Interestingly, the very mechanics meant to ensure research reliability can inadvertently perpetuate biases. Acknowledged by Peh, peer reviewers rely on reports based on information provided by authors, which can sometimes miss unconventional breakthroughs (Peh, 2021). Such scientific sieves favor orthodox approaches, even as anecdotal evidence suggests potential breakthroughs in less conventional corridors.

In preparation for exploring the forthcoming issues in conventional research, consider the scenario where enormous funding is directed toward ongoing cancer research, yet some individuals achieve remission through alternative, cost-effective means. A simple financial comparison reveals potential flaws in current research and funding priorities. The pharmaceutical economy perpetuates investments in treatments that require regular usage or provide substantial profit margins. Meanwhile, alternative treatments, despite their potential effectiveness, often lack the aggressive financial backing necessary to transition into mainstream acceptance. Highlighting these disparities invites a deeper conversation about where priorities lie and whose interests they serve.

The broader conversation requires a reimagining of both research incentives and the gatekeeping mechanisms that grant scientific legitimacy. As we turn our gaze toward the comparison of conventional financial heft against alternative successes, it's imperative to critically question whether the current model genuinely serves patient wellness or instead perpetuates an economy of dependency on certain treatments over holistic health advancements. Recognizing these biases isn't simply an academic exercise but a call to action for those dedicated to reshaping medicine's future landscape.

# The Flaws in Scientific Gatekeeping

Critics of alternative treatments often argue that these remedies lack peer review or haven't undergone rigorous clinical trials. While these concerns highlight legitimate issues of safety and efficacy, they can also serve as gatekeeping mechanisms controlled by pharmaceutical interests. This gatekeeping restricts health innovation and limits patient access to potentially beneficial therapies. The heavy influence of pharmaceutical funding complicates scientific inquiry, affecting research outcomes and public perception.

Funding sources exert substantial power over what gets studied and how results are interpreted. Conflicts of interest are especially prevalent when pharmaceutical companies finance research, generally aiming to produce results that favor their products. Such biases can stifle promising alternative treatments that don't align with industry goals or profit margins (Boden & Ozonoff, 2008). For instance, even when early stage research shows potential for alternative therapies, the lack of financial backing for large-scale clinical trials often sidelines these options. This exclusion isn't necessarily due to an absence of efficacy but rather a dearth of monetary incentive to invest in non-patentable treatments.

A poignant example is the treatment of Alzheimer's disease. Several alternative therapies have shown promise in early studies, but the lion's share of funding continues towards pharmaceutical solutions like solanezumab. This drug pursued by Eli Lilly failed to deliver meaningful results yet consumed substantial financial resources (There Are Failures, You Know, 2021). The dedication of vast amounts of money to a drug lacking clear benefit reflects a systemic preference for pharmaceutical solutions, driven by a regulatory system intertwined with industry interests.

Potentially groundbreaking alternative health approaches, like nutritional and herbal therapies, often struggle to gain traction amid such bias. The reluctance to explore these options relates less to their effectiveness and more to the absence of substantial investment for large-scale validation studies. Without the financial mark-up that comes with pharmaceuticals, these treatments often don't attract the necessary financial backing for rigorous study.

Take Vitamin D supplementation, for example, in managing a range of conditions. Peer-reviewed research supports its benefits, yet because it's inexpensive and readily available, it attracts less corporate interest for comprehensive study. Instead, research dollars pour into drugs with patent potential, sidelining affordable, readily accessible treatments with significant patient-reported success stories. This creates an ecosystem where the potential of such therapies remains underexplored, despite anecdotal evidence and smaller studies suggesting benefits.

This embedded bias affects our healthcare landscape, limiting genuine health innovation and obstructing patient access to a broad spectrum of treatments. It raises critical questions about the ethical implications of allowing financial interests to dictate medical research priorities. This structure directly impacts health freedom and patient autonomy, as individuals find themselves with limited choices driven more by market forces than by science.

For alternative health seekers and advocates of medical autonomy, such gatekeeping poses a direct challenge to individual agency. People have the right to explore and choose treatments that align with their personal beliefs and experiences. Saint John's Wort, a herb often used for depression, illustrates how regulatory gatekeeping can affect patient access. Despite evidence backing its effectiveness, its incorporation into mainstream treatment protocols remains limited. Here, the influence of existing pharmaceutical depression treatments clouds its potential widespread acceptance.

Moreover, scientific gatekeeping can affect the future of healthcare by stifling grassroots innovation. Many affordable alternative therapies emerge from individual and community experiences. When we dismiss these success stories because they lack the traditional trappings of scientific validation, we undermine the stories of real people who have improved their health through non-conventional means.

We must consider the implications of discounting personal narratives of healing in favor of expensive, sometimes ineffective pharmaceutical interventions. This choice perpetuates a cycle of financial prioritization over patient well-being, leaving individuals to navigate a convoluted healthcare system that doesn't fully serve their needs. By doing so, we risk undervaluing patient autonomy—the capacity to make informed decisions free from external pressures and undue restrictions.

Transitioning our focus toward financial priorities in health research, we face a stark contrast between the billions spent on cancer research and grassroots success stories where patients report significant improvements through affordable means. Despite extraordinary resources allocated to cancer research, some of the most compelling narratives come from those who have turned to cost-effective approaches like lifestyle changes, dietary adjustments, and complementary therapies with astounding results.

This debate challenges the conventional wisdom about resource allocation in healthcare, illuminating a landscape where patient stories might hold as much value as double-blind studies. As we move forward, it's crucial to evaluate how financial influences shape our understanding of health and well-being. These stories provide a vital counter-narrative, highlighting the possibility of health solutions that exist outside pharmaceutical frameworks.

The next challenge is evaluating these paradigms against existing scientific models. In drumming up support for diverse health approaches, it's essential to weigh patient empowerment against financial realities. This exploration shapes future discussions about fairness in research funding and the broader implications for public health strategies, setting the stage for a deeper critique of how research investment aligns—or fails to align—with meaningful patient outcomes.

# Cost Analysis of Cancer Solutions

In the previous section, we discussed the flawed logic of scientific gatekeeping, heavily influenced by pharmaceutical funding. This paradigm often determines the acceptance of medical treatments. Now, we juxtapose this with the substantial financial investments in cancer research, juxtaposed with the affordable, self-treatment successes of individuals. The mainstream medical system invests billions in research, yet many patients find relief in inexpensive, alternative solutions.

Consider the story of Jane, who turned to alternative therapies after traditional cancer treatments failed her. With a limited budget, she explored dietary changes, herbal supplements, and stress-reduction techniques. To her surprise, her condition improved significantly. Similarly, Mark, diagnosed with a terminal condition, incorporated meditation and a plant-based diet into his regimen. Despite dire predictions, he experiences a dramatic health turnaround. Their stories illustrate a pattern of unexpected success, urging us to question why mainstream medicine often ignores such alternatives.

While mainstream oncology spends upwards of USD 145,000 annually on immunotherapy for each patient (Toscano et al., 2021), patients like Jane achieve results on a fraction of that budget. More sobering are the statistics highlighting that cancer care costs could reach USD 246 billion by 2030 (Toscano et al., 2021). This stark contrast between the two approaches raises questions about the real cost-effectiveness of high-budget medical research. The discrepancy suggests that vast financial resources do not necessarily yield superior medical outcomes, a revelation that puts into question the mainstream narrative equating investment with success.

Critics argue that these financial commitments overshadow the economic simplicity of alternative treatments. When these methods lead to improved patient outcomes, the implications become profound but largely unstudied. Many patients cannot afford the skyrocketing costs of conventional cancer treatments, which may drive them towards alternative approaches. Despite evidence suggesting their potential, research into these alternatives lags significantly, primarily due to a lack of financial motivation for large corporations. If treatments lack the appeal of profitability, they're often left unexplored within the scope of traditional research frameworks.

However, this gap in research and understanding doesn't only affect patients; it reflects a significant oversight in care delivery. Financial toxicity, defined by overwhelming out-of-pocket expenses (Toscano et al., 2021), exacerbates health disparities, disproportionately affecting low-income individuals. As patients exhaust their financial resources early in their treatment journey, they face tremendous psychological and physical strain. When alternative treatments offer hope at a lower cost, ignoring them due to financial disincentives becomes ethically troubling.

Patients exploring unconventional methods often document their journeys online, sharing anecdotal evidence that reaches beyond academic journals. As they seek validation through forums, blogs, and support groups, a grassroots community emerges, united by necessity and shared experience. While skepticism of anecdotal evidence persists, the sheer breadth of these narratives demands greater academic scrutiny. These stories challenge entrenched medical assumptions, urging practitioners to reconsider the weight of subjective experiences in evidence-based medicine.

Increased scrutiny into self-treatment success might reveal significant findings otherwise obscured by focusing solely on pharmaceutical interventions. Research typically prioritizes treatments with tangible financial returns. However, the rewarding outcomes reported by patients adopting low-cost strategies shouldn't be dismissed outright. Integrating these into scientific dialogues could bridge the chasm between traditional and alternative medicines, potentially shifting treatment paradigms.

Yet, the barriers to recognizing alternative treatments extend beyond financial constraints. There's a pervasive skepticism within the medical community. Detractors often dismiss unconventional methods as placebo or impractical due to the lack of traditional empirical support. Rigorous investigation and documentation of these cases hold the potential to dispel myths surrounding them, emphasizing curiosity over cynicism.

The journey of understanding requires moving beyond conventional boundaries to rethink patient care in holistic terms. By doing so, the medical community could develop a more inclusive approach, considering alternative narratives without compromising empirical integrity. Alternative successes may complement, rather than oppose, existing medical paradigms, providing patients with more comprehensive care options.

Continued reliance on overwhelmingly costly therapies without considering economically viable alternatives further alienates patients. The pressing question becomes why the medical community doesn't demand robust investigation into the alternatives' successes. Incorporating these studies acknowledges patient-centered care, validating the diverse experiences of those navigating the healthcare system with limited means.

The need for change calls for extensive dialogue, encouraging collaboration between traditional practitioners and advocates of alternative treatments. Facilitating open communication and sharing knowledge will dismantle existing silos. By approaching case studies like Jane's and Mark's with scientific rigor, we could unlock new insights into efficacious, affordable treatment models.

Ultimately, the crux of this discussion highlights a critical examination of our priorities in healthcare research and delivery. The trajectory towards universally accessible, affordable healthcare grows clearer through reconciling mainstream and alternative approaches. By re-evaluating the way we assess treatment success, nuanced insights from individual experiences could inspire transformative change.

The reality of financial constraints faced by patients illustrates an urgent need to transcend traditional medical perspectives. Embracing innovative, patient-centered approaches presents an overdue opportunity for the medical community to expand its paradigms of healing. Responsible, ethical healthcare research includes examining low-cost, effective methods, ensuring every patient has access to the highest quality care without financial ruin.

# Final Thoughts

In closing this chapter, we've delved into the persistent challenges faced by alternative treatments in a world dominated by pharmaceutical interests. It's clear that mainstream medicine often overlooks these methods, not due to ineffectiveness but because they don't fit within the profit-driven framework. However, as more individuals share their success stories and seek autonomy over their health choices, the demand for broader acceptance and integration of these alternatives grows louder. Now that we understand the layered reasons behind this oversight, we can push for a future where healthcare embraces diverse healing methods, valuing patient experiences alongside traditional evidence. By doing so, we pave the way for a medical landscape that truly prioritizes holistic well-being over financial gain, encouraging an inclusive approach that acknowledges all viable paths to health.

# Chapter 8 The Pattern of Suppression

If Lisa's success with her unconventional health treatments surprised some, it downright enraged others. For years, she had been dismissed by conventional doctors, who insisted that alternative methods weren't backed by "real science." Yet, the anecdotal evidence was hard to ignore. Friends and family members saw their ailments improve after following Lisa's advice, which included dietary changes and natural supplements that mainstream medicine often scoffed at. Despite the skeptics, her community of patients steadily grew, many of them desperate for relief after traditional treatments had failed them.

The question remains: why do these alternate paths continue to face such fierce resistance from established medical systems, especially when so many people report seeing improvements? In this chapter, we'll delve into the reasons behind the skepticism that mainstream medicine holds towards alternative treatments. We will explore how financial interests and institutional biases shape which therapies are given credibility—and why some like Lisa's, despite showing promise, remain on the fringe. Does the medical world have room for both approaches, or is its reluctance keeping potential solutions hidden in the shadows?

# Lisa's Journey and Introduction and Avoidance by Mainstream Medicine

Scientific gatekeeping in healthcare often raises questions about the interplay of economic forces and research priorities. Financial influences profoundly influence the perceived legitimacy of treatments, often sidelining alternative therapies. Looking at the mechanisms through which financial interests prevail can unravel biases in how medical research prioritizes conventional over alternative treatments. Such biases manifest largely because of the pervasive profit-driven agendas in mainstream medicine, effectively determining which therapies get the spotlight and which remain in the shadows.

Big pharmaceutical companies are significant stakeholders in this paradigm, with considerable resources directed toward promoting conventional treatments. Their financial might allows them to fund extensive research, clinical trials, and marketing campaigns to consolidate their market position. In contrast, alternative therapies often lack similar resources. Consequently, they miss out on comprehensive studies that could validate their efficacy (Mortada, 2024; Ventola, 2010). This financial imbalance creates a knowledge gap, influencing guidelines about treatment safety and efficacy. Clinicians rely on such research-backed data to make patient care decisions, and without comparable data for alternative treatments, these therapies find less acceptance in mainstream practice.

The systemic bias against alternative treatments is further amplified by the close nexus between pharmaceutical companies and regulatory bodies. Such entities wield substantial control over the research agenda, often prioritizing studies that promise financial returns over those aligning with broader patient-centered outcomes. Dr. Johanna Budwig's case provides a poignant example. Despite her groundbreaking work in developing cancer treatments that showed promise, she faced dismissal because her theories did not align with conventional scientific understanding or pharmaceutical profit models. Her therapies, which emphasized natural dietary changes, ran counter to the established drug-centric approaches, leaving them unsupported by large research funds (Mortada, 2024).

Scientific journals also play a role in perpetuating this bias. Peer review, a crucial part of determining research credibility, often marginalizes studies focusing on alternative treatments. These journals tend to favor research with robust funding and methodologies derived from conventional approaches. As a result, many alternative therapies lack representation in reputable journals, further skewing the evidence landscape. Given that clinicians and medical professionals routinely consult these journals to stay updated, the paucity of studies supporting alternative treatments stunts their integration into mainstream practices (Ventola, 2010).

The prioritization of research funding also reflects broader societal biases concerning the value of alternative therapies. Cultural perceptions often paint alternative medicine as less scientific or credible than mainstream treatments. The lack of rigorous scientific validation perpetuates this stereotype, despite considerable anecdotal evidence of their efficacy and calls for integrative approaches that combine the best of both worlds (Mortada, 2024). These overarching narratives significantly shape healthcare policies and, consequently, how alternative treatments are perceived and utilized in patient care.

Public health systems, influenced by pharmaceutical lobbying, further uphold this imbalance by investing heavily in conventional medicine. This patronage ensures that new pharmaceutical treatments swiftly travel from research to clinical application, ensuring continued financial growth for these companies. However, it leaves alternative therapies struggling to navigate bureaucratic hurdles. In countries where integrative approaches have gained ground, such steps are often driven by grassroots advocacy and consumer demand rather than institutional support (Mortada, 2024; Ventola, 2010).

Patients, frustrated with the limitations of conventional medicine, increasingly turn to alternative therapies, seeking holistic treatments that address their needs. This consumer-driven demand reveals a disconnect between institutional priorities and patient preferences. However, the absence of significant research hinders these patients from making informed decisions. Given the ethical duty to provide patient-centered care, healthcare systems must reevaluate how they determine the legitimacy and integration of treatments, considering both scientific evidence and patient satisfaction (Mortada, 2024).

Moving forward, challenging these biases requires a shift in how research is approached and funded. Cross-disciplinary collaborations can facilitate integrative studies that explore the confluence of conventional and alternative medicine. Such collaborative research efforts would provide a more comprehensive understanding of treatment efficacy and safety. Incentives for researchers aiming to bridge this gap could stimulate interest in exploring alternative medicines, leading to a broader acceptance of diverse treatment modalities in clinical practice.

The financial challenges facing alternative therapies often lead to their dismissal by mainstream medicine. Alternative practitioners frequently find themselves marginalized, their treatments dismissed as lacking evidence. The next section will delve into how financial dynamics constrain these therapies, exploring how mainstream medicine's economic interests shape the modern medical landscape. By examining concrete examples of dismissed therapies and sidelined practitioners, we'll understand the broader consequences for patient care and the necessary steps to redress these imbalances.

Ultimately, redefining research prioritization requires dismantling financial and cultural biases ingrained within the scientific gatekeeping process. Health systems must commit to patient-focused care, where the value of integrative approaches is recognized and supported, ensuring that prescriptions and treatments are genuinely in patients' best interests. Such reform would not only validate the significance of alternative therapies but also acknowledge the complexities of modern patient needs.

# Traditional Criticisms Analyzed

The last section dissected the flawed logic behind scientific gatekeeping, where restrictive, conventional frameworks undermine alternative medicine's credibility. Financial interests frequently dictate what treatments gain acceptance. This theme manifests in Jane and Mark's stories as they navigate health interventions that challenge mainstream medical skepticism.

For Jane, plagued by chronic pain and frustrated by her expensive mainstream treatments, alternative medicine offered a relief conventional methods failed to provide. Faced with mounting medical bills for therapies that only moderately alleviated her symptoms, Jane turned to options dismissed by her primary care physician. Acupuncture and massage therapy became her salvation, offering more substantial, enduring relief at a fraction of the cost of her monthly prescriptions (Fønnebø et al., 2007). Jane's story illuminates the critical point that a disconnect persists between costly conventional medical practices and the overlooked efficacy of alternative treatments. Her experience suggests that health improvements needn't correlate with expense, thus challenging the narrative that a therapy's financial backing equates to effectiveness.

Similarly, Mark's battle with stress-induced migraines paints a vivid picture of potential missed opportunities in conventional medicine. As a successful ad executive, Mark could afford the customary medical interventions prescribed, yet they yielded little improvement. However, upon integrating cost-effective complementary methods such as biofeedback and guided imagery, Mark found significant relief that existing prescriptions couldn't match (Herman et al., 2005). His positive outcomes without the need for costly pharmaceuticals demonstrate an essential reconsideration of the entrenched idea that legitimacy in medicine requires hefty investments and financial interest. Mark's journey compels us to question why low-cost, high-value approaches remain underutilized.

Their stories illustrate broader notions about the financial hegemony within healthcare systems. Pharmaceutical companies notoriously invest in extensive campaigns that bolster their treatments' credibility, often overshadowing lesser-funded innovations. By juxtaposing Jane and Mark's cost-efficient triumphs with mainstream medicine's high-priced endorsements, these individual victories advocate for a reexamination of health research's economic focus. Their experiences serve as palpable case studies advocating for alternative medicine's integration into the discourse, advancing the argument for a significant shift in healthcare priorities that value clinical outcomes over financial clout.

Jane and Mark's paths further reveal that dismissing alternative treatments collectively due to limited randomized clinical trial endorsements misses the individual stories where these therapies excel. Both found that therapies commonly labeled as unproven or dubious by conventional gatekeepers provided marked improvements. This positions their stories as counterweights in the ongoing debate on efficacy versus financial investment, encouraging skepticism towards equating financial prowess with therapeutic legitimacy. Mainstream health systems must evolve to recognize successful low-cost alternatives without being tethered to prevailing economic interests.

These personal accounts point to a paradigm where financial incentives potentially obscure valuable, affordable treatments. A significant aspect of this issue arises when mainstream healthcare and medical professionals disregard personal testimonies due to a lack of statistically significant, large-scale trials. However, Jane and Mark's enhanced wellbeing offers powerful evidence warranting the reevaluation of mainstream medicine's dismissive tendencies toward unvetted alternatives (Fønnebø et al., 2007). Highlighting how generic pain relievers and upscale prescriptions starkly contrast with the effective simplicity of acupuncture or biofeedback promotes an essential critique that existing healthcare models insufficiently prioritize meaningful patient outcomes.

Moreover, retracing the nuances of these personal tales underscores the blind spots embedded within the healthcare research infrastructure. Patients like Jane and Mark turn towards alternatives when conventional systems fall short, primarily due to limited alternative treatment evaluations and inconsistent funding. Their stories serve as a clarion call, not only advocating for increased research into alternative treatment modalities but effectively querying the motives guiding current healthcare investment strategies (Herman et al., 2005). The overarching need demands robust frameworks that reliably integrate patient-owned narratives as valid evidence, from which both current and prospective research angles might expand.

Continuing down this path directs focus towards financial determinants obfuscating genuine choice in healthcare, hence steering narratives like Jane's and Mark's into the spotlight to reframe understanding and acceptance of complementary therapies. Leveraging these insights sets the foundation for the next section to explore systemic impact and reveals how financial motivations influence patient autonomy and innovation integrity. This thriller-like intrigue of patient independence versus institutional dominion propels us forward, promising a deep dive into ethical considerations and health equity progression.

Insightful exploration of the key narratives, woven with conviction and evidence, implores a shift in understanding how medicine equates cost to care. Stories of individual success amidst financial and institutional resistance summon a new outlook on treatment validation, one where monetary influence must yield to diverse innovation and comprehensive human experiences. As we examine the wider impacts, the challenge remains to prioritize authenticity over economics in the shaping of future health paradigms.

# The Flaws in Scientific Gatekeeping and Cost Analysis of Cancer Solutions

In our earlier analysis, we unveiled how scientific gatekeeping backed by pharmaceutical funding often skews the research landscape. This starter sheds light on the barriers posed by financial interests that limit the scope of innovative alternative treatments in healthcare. These systemic obstructions not only maintain the status quo but also prevent patients from accessing potentially life-saving alternative therapies. Reflecting on this, one has to wonder: why, despite their potential, do these treatments struggle for legitimacy in mainstream medicine?

The dominance of financial interests in healthcare research leads to a prioritization that favors treatments providing substantial returns. This financial inclination influences the choice of research topics, often sidelining therapies with little or no profitability, even if they show potential benefits. In many cases, interest groups dictate research agendas, colors the understanding of treatment efficacy and narrows the available choices for patients navigating their health journeys. For instance, Dr. Johanna Budwig's dietary protocol, which emphasizes healthy fats and a natural diet over conventional cancer treatments, struggles to gain traction primarily due to a lack of financial motivation to fund comprehensive studies. Similarly, laetrile, derived from apricot pits and proposed for cancer treatment, ignites controversy partly because large pharmaceutical companies cannot patent or profit significantly from its use, creating a roadblock to its investigation and possible integration into accepted practices.

While anecdotal success stories provide glimpses of these therapies' potential, they often remain unrecognized in clinical settings. The traditional research model, driven largely by profit, overlooks countless instances where patients benefit from alternative treatments. Such an oversight points to a significant disconnect between real-world success stories and clinical practice. Some patients who have turned to unconventional therapies when standard treatments failed report promising outcomes. Yet, without meaningful financial incentives, research exploring these methods lacks the robust funding required to propel them into the mainstream medical discourse.

Patient autonomy should allow individuals the freedom to explore all potential treatments. However, with financial interests regularly steering the ship, market forces ultimately shape healthcare priorities and options. The ethical implications of this are profound. Patients should feel empowered, choosing treatments that align with their values and experiences rather than having their options constrained by the economic interests of powerful entities. The recurring theme illustrates how financial motivations restrict patient autonomy, an obstacle to achieving a more inclusive healthcare model.

Nonetheless, community narratives and grassroots movements offer a different kind of power. These stories, often dismissed as mere anecdotes, challenge established evidence-based frameworks and introduce a new layer to the discourse about alternative treatments. They possess the potential to shift perspectives and ignite wider conversations about healthcare choices. These narratives empower individuals and communities, fueling movements that advocate for recognition and integration of alternative therapies. In doing so, they help balance the concentrated scientific power, urging the healthcare system to reconsider overlooked options.

For example, many individuals share their experiences with cannabis-based treatments for chronic pain—stories initially brushed aside but now gaining recognition as cannabis finds its way into more mainstream avenues. As these stories become louder, grassroots organizations advocate for legislative changes and broader acceptance, succeeding in setting the stage for more comprehensive discussions on treatment accessibility.

Onward, we approach exploration of individual and community successes with alternative therapies. It's essential to highlight how these stories not only contribute to personal health narratives but also advocate for their inclusion in broader scientific research. As this exploration grows, so does the call for integrating patient-centered care models that accommodate diverse treatment approaches. These narratives question the traditional scientific approach, demanding inclusion in research and illustrating that financial and scientific constraints need not be unyielding barriers.

As we delve further into these community-driven successes, there's a need to frame the dialogue within the context of transitioning from financial constraints to universal healthcare access. This transition is crucial to ensuring that patients receive care tailored to their needs, beyond the confines of financially-driven medical models. By doing so, the healthcare system not only becomes more inclusive but also embraces a spirit of adaptability—responding to the diverse and evolving needs of patients.

In summary, the discussion on the intertwining of financial interests with medical research and treatment availability reinforces a necessity for change. By examining real-world stories and recognizing the role of grassroots movements, there's an opportunity to reshape healthcare discourse. As healthcare systems evolve, they will need to accommodate a diversity of voices and experiences, ultimately fostering an environment that values patient autonomy and diverse treatment pathways. It is a call for a healthcare paradigm that goes beyond profitability, honoring the full spectrum of healing possibilities that exist within alternative treatments.

In the ongoing dialogue about healthcare, the entrenched skepticism of mainstream medicine towards alternative health treatments stands as a notable barrier to their broader acceptance. Central to this issue is the logic of scientific gatekeeping, which often dictates what is deemed legitimate within the medical community. Scientific gatekeeping insists on rigorous evidence standards, typically defined by clinical trials and peer-reviewed research, which many alternative therapies lack due to limited funding and structural biases (Ross, 2009). The pharmaceutical industry plays a significant role in shaping these standards, as their funding heavily influences the direction of medical research. Substantial financial resources allow pharmaceuticals to conduct comprehensive research and secure regulatory approval, creating a pipeline that naturally slants towards their products. Alternative health treatments, without the backing of similar capital, struggle to meet these arbitrary benchmarks, limiting their acceptance and integration into mainstream practices.

Financial biases extend beyond research funding. The intricate web of healthcare operations, encompassing insurance companies and healthcare providers, often sidelines alternative treatments. Insurance policies frequently don't cover these therapies, leaving patients to incur out-of-pocket expenses. This not only reduces access but perpetuates the narrative that alternative treatments lack credibility (Mortada, 2024). The integration of these treatments remains elusive, obstructed by financial dynamics designed around conventional medicine. In this economic climate, alternative health modalities face an uphill battle for legitimacy, pigeonholed as supplementary rather than complementary.

Yet, patient experiences paint a different picture. Individuals like Jane and Mark illustrate how alternative therapies can significantly improve personal health and well-being. Jane, struggling with chronic pain unresponsive to medications, explored acupuncture. Her self-reported improvements herald a broader narrative of effectiveness that isn't captured in traditional clinical trials. Similarly, Mark's journey with herbal remedies for anxiety underscores the potential for non-pharmaceutical interventions. These stories reverberate with audiences seeking natural, holistic health solutions that emphasize personal health autonomy. For many, these treatments are not an either-or choice but a both/and addition to conventional treatments. They thrive in the gray area, offering relief where mainstream medicine may falter.

Mainstream medicine, rooted in evidence-based practices, often overlooks such anecdotal successes. Evidence-based medicine, as defined, depends on quantifiable data from systematic research (Mortada, 2024). This dependency underscores a critical challenge: not all healing is quantifiable by current scientific standards. The experiences of those like Jane and Mark challenge the status quo, arguing for a reformed understanding of evidence that values both traditional data and personal testimony. Practitioners rooted in evidence-based medicine must recognize the credibility in these patient narratives. While anecdotal evidence shouldn't replace scientific research, it merits a role in shaping an inclusive healthcare model that aligns with patient needs and preferences (Ross, 2009).

Critics assert that bypassing rigorous evidence risks patient safety. Their concerns are valid; safety and efficacy remain paramount. But the inflexible application of these criteria fails to accommodate emerging healing modalities that prioritize patient empowerment and autonomy. Patients increasingly want control over their health decisions, preferring personalized approaches over one-size-fits-all models. Alternative treatments offer this, fostering an environment that honors individual preference and cultural diversity.

The success stories of holistic and cost-effective solutions not only validate alternative therapies but pressure a reevaluation of medical dismissiveness. These therapies, ranging from simple lifestyle adjustments to complex integrative practices, provide cost-effective options that resonate in a climate of high medical expenses. Economic accessibility is a compelling argument for their broader acceptance. By easing financial burdens, these treatments encourage patients to explore comprehensive, sustainable health strategies. As patients report improved outcomes with these alternatives, the demand for their integration into mainstream healthcare systems mounts.

Such integration would benefit not just patients. Healthcare practitioners stand to gain from a diversified toolset, enhancing their ability to deliver holistic care (Mortada, 2024). This evolution enriches the healthcare continuum, embracing a model that appreciates the interplay of body, mind, and spirit in health and healing. From the perspective of policy, embracing alternative medicine requires an openness to evolving definitions of efficacy. Regulatory frameworks need adaptation, ensuring they account for diverse forms of evidence and celebrate the multifaceted nature of healing.

Regulatory oversight can facilitate safe usage, addressing skepticism with rigorous yet accessible pathways for validation. By incorporating diverse healing methods into healthcare systems, we address demographic shifts towards integrative medicine, responding to a market that increasingly demands these alternatives. This step requires courage from both practitioners and policymakers to evaluate entrenched beliefs and biases (Ross, 2009). It necessitates policy that supports research funding, guided not by pharmaceutical interests but by genuine inquiry into complementary and alternative therapies. By fostering such environments, we create a landscape where diverse treatment modalities coexist, meeting the nuanced needs of global populations.

Confronting the financial and institutional biases limiting alternative health treatments remains a formidable challenge. Yet, as Jane's and Mark's narratives demonstrate, these therapies hold undeniable promise and potential. Calls for broader acceptance aren't just about integrating alternative medicine; they resonate with deeper values of personal autonomy, patient empowerment, and comprehensive care. Moving beyond rhetoric, it's time for healthcare systems to adopt this broader vision, weaving alternative and complementary treatments into a fabric that honors both their potential and humanity's intricate dance between evidence and experience. Addressing these challenges proactively fosters a future where healthcare is not just about curing disease but nurturing wellness in every dimension.

## Final Thoughts

Now that we understand the entrenched skepticism of mainstream medicine toward alternative treatments, it becomes clearer why these therapies face significant challenges. Driven by monetary interests and scientific gatekeeping, mainstream systems often overlook the real-life successes of countless individuals who turn to alternatives when traditional methods fail them. With their stories in mind, it's vital for the future of healthcare to embrace diverse healing practices, integrating them into conventional frameworks. This integration isn't just about broadening the scope of available treatments; it's about honoring patient autonomy, empowering individuals with more choices, and ensuring that healing is approached holistically. By prioritizing both rigorous research and personal narratives, health systems can evolve to meet the complex needs of today's patients, encouraging a more inclusive and adaptable medical landscape.

# Chapter 9 RFK Jr., Autism, and the War on Truth

Have you ever found yourself questioning the truth behind medical advice that seems to change with every new study or emerging health scare? It's a confusing landscape, one where skepticism may feel like the only constant companion. Robert F. Kennedy Jr. knows this feeling all too well. His journey through the murky waters of modern medicine highlights the challenges faced by anyone daring to voice dissent. As RFK Jr. speaks on topics like autism diagnoses and mRNA vaccines, he faces pushback not unlike what we've seen with historical figures who challenged the status quo in their time.

Imagine navigating a world where your perspective is constantly under fire, not just in terms of disagreement but with accusations that extend to being dangerous. This chapter dives into how figures like RFK Jr. are often portrayed, exploring the mechanisms behind media narratives that simplify complex issues into polars of right and wrong. We'll look closer at the rise in autism diagnoses post-COVID-19 and consider how dissenting voices in medicine can inform this dialogue. As the chapter unfolds, we'll go beyond headlines to understand the intricacies of medical debates, from vaccine opposition to autism statistics, seeking to illuminate the paths forward for those who dare to question established norms.

# Introduction of RFK Jr.'s Challenges and Parallels with Clark's Persecution

Robert F. Kennedy Jr.'s journey has been marked by struggles and scrutiny, reminiscent of historical figures who challenged convention in their time. He faces intense public and media criticism, primarily for his outspoken views on autism diagnoses and mRNA vaccines. RFK Jr.'s experience aligns with a broader narrative where dissenting voices in medicine encounter fierce opposition, often being labeled "dangerous." This framework isn't new—historical figures like Nobel laureate Linus Pauling, who advocated for high-dose vitamin C as a cancer treatment, initially faced backlash from his peers for crossing the boundaries of traditional medicine. They, too, challenged prevailing beliefs, often meeting resistance before their ideas gained wider acceptance.

In examining RFK Jr.'s case, it's essential to consider the nuances of media portrayal and the impact of public scrutiny. The vilification often overshadows the substance of his arguments, reducing complex issues to binary debates. The media, in its quest for compelling narratives, may emphasize controversy over nuanced discourse. This echoes how societal narratives can polarize public opinion, much like the historical example of Clarence Darrow's defense in the Scopes "Monkey" Trial, where scientific inquiry clashed with entrenched beliefs about evolution and education.

RFK Jr.'s advocacy against mRNA vaccines is particularly contentious, as it challenges powerful pharmaceutical narratives. It draws parallels to the skepticism faced by Ignaz Semmelweis, who advocated for hand-washing among doctors to prevent childbed fever—an idea that met harsh criticism at the time. Like Semmelweis, RFK Jr. contends with skepticism and resistance, serving as a reminder of the friction often faced by those challenging established norms. In both cases, the impetus is to protect public health, albeit through avenues not universally embraced.

The public's response to medical dissent often mirrors broader societal discomfort with ambiguity and change. We're reminded of Robert Moses's influence in reshaping New York's infrastructure, which in turn impacted access for diverse communities (Schindler, 2015). Moses's actions highlight how powerful figures can affect societal structures, paralleling how influential narratives in medicine shape public perception and policy. The interplay between power, public health, and the accessibility of diverse perspectives frames the challenges faced by those like RFK Jr.

Furthermore, Kennedy's plight isn't isolated to his criticism of vaccines. His efforts coincide with rising autism diagnoses, creating a perfect storm of controversy post-COVID-19. Social dynamics often amplify tensions between dissenting voices and institutional stances, akin to the story of infrastructure decisions in Atlanta, Georgia, where public transit development faced opposition, perpetuating barriers for communities of color (Schindler, 2015). These are not merely stories of physical barriers but reflect how societal boundaries reinforce existing divides, much like the rigid narratives surrounding medical dissent.

In exploring RFK Jr.'s journey, his commitment to truth and transparency underscores the complexities of grappling with scientific evolution. Just as Rachel Carson faced criticism for her work in environmental science, RFK Jr.'s journey exemplifies the ongoing struggle between established paradigms and the necessity for open dialogue in emerging scientific questions. Carson's advocacy—eventually recognized for its monumental impact—parallels Kennedy's pursuit of what he perceives as a broader medical truth.

Criticism directed at RFK Jr. frequently revolves around his approach, painting him as an antivaccine activist rather than delving into the substance of his arguments. The need for balanced discussion in media narratives mirrors the exploration of social dynamics in Memphis, where infrastructure changes underscored racial divides, as illustrated by the deliberate street closures to separate communities (Schindler, 2015). The perceived threat of differing views often becomes a reflection of deeper societal fears, much like the simmering tensions in urban planning that reinforce societal stratifications.

Kennedy's message resonates with audiences seeking alternative health solutions, who challenge mainstream narratives. His supporters, akin to citizens advocating for expanded public transit options in urban areas (Schindler, 2015), reflect the continuous push for inclusivity and diversity in healthcare narratives. Yet, like historical urban planning decisions excluding certain populations (Bukar, 2020), entrenched systems often favor established structures over innovative, albeit contentious, proposals.

As RFK Jr. navigates this complex landscape, he embodies the spirit of historical figures who dared to confront prevailing beliefs. His struggle illuminates the enduring friction between established perspectives and emerging voices in complex dialogues. The reluctance to engage with dissent through constructive conversation often sidelines valuable insights, potentially delaying progress in understanding intricate medical phenomena like the rising autism rates post-pandemic.

The path forward requires open dialogue, transcending simplified narratives to embrace a spectrum of perspectives. Just as historical debates on infrastructure and urban planning have revealed societal stratifications, the discourse surrounding RFK Jr.'s advocacy must engage with diverse viewpoints. As this chapter segues into the statistical analysis of autism diagnoses since COVID-19's onset, understanding these dynamics is crucial. The upcoming discussion will delve into potential causes, societal impacts, and ongoing debates within the medical community. In doing so, it seeks to provide clarity on an issue that, much like RFK Jr.'s journey, requires a nuanced, inclusive approach.

# The Rise in Autism Diagnoses Post-COVID-19

The journey of Robert F. Kennedy Jr. grappling with contentious discussions is emblematic of a broader contention involving autism and post-pandemic diagnoses. As we delve into the nuances of increased autism diagnoses following COVID-19, striking parallels emerge between these debates. Kennedy Jr.'s challenges foreground a tapestry of complexity where perceptions and scientific evidence often clash, reflecting similar dynamics in understanding autism today. This section endeavors not only to dissect statistical trends but also to unravel underlying narratives that define the contemporary discourse on autism.

Following COVID-19, a notable uptick in autism diagnoses has captured attention, demanding a nuanced exploration of associated causes and impacts. Data pointing to increased diagnoses reflects a multifaceted puzzle, influenced by altered environmental and societal conditions post-pandemic. The surge in autism cases might partly stem from diagnostic shifts as heightened awareness led to more screenings and subsequent identifications. Simultaneously, the pervasive disruption of routines and stability during the pandemic might have exacerbated symptoms indistinguishable from autism, contributing to the increase in diagnoses (Dal Pai et al., 2022).

The social and educational repercussions of this uptick create a ripple effect, extending the challenges faced by families and institutions. Caregivers experience amplified strain navigating complex healthcare and educational systems not equipped for sudden influxes of special needs cases. The pandemic-induced isolation disturbed conventional support networks, amplifying existing hurdles (Baweja et al., 2021). Many families confront profound uncertainty, grappling with services shortages and inconsistent access to essential therapies—an echo of Brookes et al.'s (2020) findings on increased psychological burdens during crises.

Exploring these societal impacts further, one observes how educational frameworks struggle under pressure. Schools attempt to accommodate larger numbers of students with autism, reshaping instructional techniques and resource allocation. These institutions often lack sufficient personnel trained in special education, exacerbating the challenge. Children with autism, thus, face inconsistencies in learning environments, affecting their academic and social development. The necessity for adaptable and inclusive education becomes ever more apparent as schools endeavor to meet diverse needs (Baweja et al., 2021).

Within the medical community, fierce debates ensue over the nature and implications of rising autism diagnoses. Some professionals argue that pandemic-related stressors and heightened vigilance contribute to the statistical spike. Others propose that evolving diagnostic criteria accommodate the spectrum's breadth, capturing more cases without necessarily indicating an actual increase in prevalence (Dal Pai et al., 2022). This dichotomy prompts further exploration of autism's etiology and expression, challenging existing paradigms while fostering robust scientific dialogue.

Concrete examples from health forums highlight divergent perspectives on what constitutes autism and how it manifests. These anecdotal insights, backed by Eshraghi et al. (2020), illuminate the lived experiences of families whose journeys through medical systems mirror larger societal struggles. Individuals recount stories of delayed interventions and misdiagnoses pre-pandemic, showing a long-standing need for systemic reform heightened by current circumstances.

Critically, this discourse intersects with broader themes of health disparity, as examined by Kullar et al. (2020). Historically marginalized communities experience disproportionate impacts, where barriers to healthcare access exacerbate autism diagnosis challenges. The pandemic's legacy on societal inequities reveals persistent gaps. When intersected with autism diagnoses, these disparities demand comprehensive strategies to ensure equitable healthcare provision.

Underpinning the medical community's ongoing debate is the broader context of how dissent and diverse viewpoints contribute to medical advancement. Autism's complexity exemplifies the need for varied perspectives enhancing understanding and treatment. As the community faces these challenges, open dialogue becomes crucial, reconciling differing opinions to advance a more inclusive model of care and understanding.

The transition from discussing autism's increased diagnoses to upcoming debates on mRNA vaccines provides a tangible connection between personal, medical, and societal realms. Here, the intricacies of autism intersect with broader medical discourses, where dissenting views and skepticism about scientific consensus remain central. Exploring the impacts of mRNA vaccine opposition exemplifies a continuation of examining how credible dissent shapes and challenges prevailing narratives.

In preparing to delve into vaccine discourse, one discerns intersecting threads of truth-seeking and skepticism, reflecting broader societal currents. As we explore the implications of vaccine opposition, RFK Jr.'s experiences underscore a persistent theme of questioning authority while navigating controversial scientific landscapes. This transition, while contextualizing autism's practical and theoretical impacts, sets the stage for analyzing how vaccines, trust, and public health narratives intertwine.

These developments portray an evolving narrative of both challenge and opportunity. Autism diagnoses post-COVID-19 illuminate broader societal tensions while fostering critical examination within scientific and public spheres. Engaging this ongoing dialogue marks a step towards shifting paradigms, where embracing multifaceted perspectives reshapes approaches to health, truth, and understanding.

# Opposition to mRNA Vaccines and Censorship Issues

The rise in autism diagnoses during and after the COVID-19 pandemic presents a complex issue intertwined with ongoing debates about mRNA vaccines and the marginalization of dissident medical voices. This pattern underscores a larger narrative about how dissent within the scientific community is often deemed 'dangerous,' both by societal standards and prevailing scientific establishments. Dissent, in this context, isn't necessarily a divisive force. Instead, it could offer renewed perspectives necessary for authentic scientific progress and public health betterment.

When we address dissent in medical and scientific fields, it's crucial to examine how established institutions and mainstream media shape public perceptions. These entities frequently frame dissident voices as threats, rather than constructive challenges to prevailing norms. This framing often results in a narrative that discourages critical examination and stifles open dialogue. The contention around mRNA vaccines, which integrate new technology with inconclusive testing results (Wallis, 2023), serves as a pertinent example. Dissenting doctors who proposed alternative treatments were censured, highlighting the delicate landscape that challenges current medical dogmas.

The case of Dr. Aseem Malhotra exemplifies the intricate relationship between dissent and perceived danger. Initially an advocate for vaccines, Dr. Malhotra reversed his stance, citing concerns over myocarditis risks, which Pfizer itself acknowledged (Wallis, 2023). His journey sparked a shift in opinions, revealing the potential hazards when dissenting voices are dismissed outright. The labeling of dissent in this manner often hinges on an assumption: that any deviation from mainstream science could disrupt public trust in essential health interventions. This tension becomes a tug-of-war between safeguarding public health and fostering innovation through diversity of thought.

Dissenting voices like those of Dr. Robert V. Malone and Peter McCullough offer narratives that resist quick dismissal. Their concerns about vaccine safety and the impact of chronic illnesses on COVID-19 vulnerabilities uncover gaps in health systems sometimes overlooked in public discourse

(Wallis, 2023). Reverberating through their arguments is the notion that labeling dissent as dangerous risks stagnation in scientific understanding. It discourages examination of potentially significant variables, such as the long-term effects of rapidly developed medical interventions.

Moreover, historical examples, like the case of Dr. Andrew Wakefield, caution against premature repudiations. Dr. Wakefield's early inquiries into the MMR vaccine and autism, although controversial, emphasize the dangers of conflating inquiry with falsehood (Wallis, 2023). Misinterpretations of his work and the subsequent revocation of his medical license highlight how punitive measures against medical dissent can stifle future investigations, regardless of merit. This response reflects broader societal tendencies to obscure dissent under a veil of threat rather than a potential source of new insight.

The societal labeling of dissent as dangerous extends beyond the medical field into public and political realms. This dynamic influences policy formation and skews health strategies towards predominantly accepted viewpoints. In the case of the COVID-19 response, the purported threat posed by dissent swayed the public towards skepticism about alternative narratives. This reactionary stance risks limiting access to potentially lifesaving strategies that deviate from mainstream protocols.

To counteract the marginalization of dissent while maintaining public trust, and informed policy-making, a reimagined approach is necessary. First, promoting a cultural shift towards valuing diverse scientific opinions could expand the breadth of examined data, advanced hypotheses, and tested theories. Validating dissent can lead to a robust verification process, as opposed to mere conflict. When scrutinizing the narratives around COVID-19 vaccines, for example, encouragement of comprehensive research into reported adverse effects and vaccine efficiency could lend critical depth to public health discussions (Igyártó & Qin, 2024).

Furthermore, transparency and active engagement are instrumental in reshaping the conversation. Open forums where divergent views on public health can be debated constructively offer a platform for scientists who contest prevailing assumptions to express ideas without fear of censorship. Media and health authorities could bridge gaps between acceptance of innovative dissent and maintenance of public safety.

Ultimately, the sociopolitical reach of scientific and medical dissent, as delineated within today's society, raises pertinent concerns about the systemic practice of labeling dissent as inherently dangerous. Counteracting this commonplace practice does more than encourage a well-rounded scientific debate; it enhances scientific creativity and responsiveness to unforeseen challenges, reflecting positively on collective health outcomes.

As public discourse evolves, it's important to reiterate that dissent should serve as a catalyst, not just a conflict point. Encouraging a culture that celebrates intellectual diversity not only aligns with democratic ideals but enhances the potential for scientific progress. The next dialogue chapter will explore further the evolving conversation around encouraging open scientific inquiry, delving into how reframing dissent can lead to more resilient, inclusive, and innovative public health landscapes.

# Framing Dissent in Medicine as 'Dangerous'

In the earlier discussion about mRNA vaccine opposition, we noted how dissenting opinions can be quickly marginalized. This marginalization exemplifies a broader tendency to label medical dissent as dangerous, effectively stifling meaningful dialogue and potential breakthroughs. In the realm of medicine, dissent is often demonized, resulting in a chilling effect that discourages open inquiry and innovation.

Indeed, those who express concerns about mRNA vaccines or any other controversial topics in medicine often find themselves battling against this pejorative labeling. The argument, as de Melo-Martín and Intemann explain, is that labeling dissent as problematic ignores the essential role this discourse plays in driving scientific advancement (de Melo-Martín & Intemann, 2012). By branding dissent as dangerous, particularly in the complex and vital field of medicine, we run the risk of dismissing voices that may offer vital insights or highlight overlooked aspects of prevailing theories.

The negative framing of medical dissent has its roots in the way dissenters are perceived as threats to public health and policy. As Nash points out, targeting dissent is seen by some as a protective measure against misinformation and its potential dangers (Nash, 2018). This perspective suggests that blocking dissent may prevent harm. However, this approach fails to address the underlying causes, such as the public's misunderstanding of scientific complexities, which strengthens the noise of dissenting voices that aim not at contributing but at creating doubt.

Examples throughout history show how this suppression of diverse views can hinder progress. Consider the early debates on the heliocentric model of the solar system. Initial dissent against the geocentric view paved the way for scientific breakthroughs that transformed humanity's understanding of the universe. Yet, dissenters like Galileo faced severe backlash, including charges of heresy. These historical instances provide lessons relevant today: stifling dissent in medicine could mean missing out on groundbreaking discoveries that originate from unconventional ideas.

What's more, perceptions of dissent as dangerous can be reinforced by media misinterpretations and political agendas that oversimplify scientific nuances. Media portrayals often simplify complex studies into catchy headlines that misrepresent the findings, compounding public misunderstanding. As de Melo-Martín and Intemann observed, when disagreements are misinterpreted, it can lead to a skewed perception that results in misinformed policy decisions (de Melo-Martín & Intemann, 2012).

Addressing dissent more constructively involves encouraging a paradigm shift in how dissenters are viewed. Instead of instinctively dismissing dissent, it would be more constructive to foster environments where diverse opinions are dissected and debated with rigor and openness. This approach is especially crucial in medicine, where innovation often comes from challenging established norms. Cultivating a culture that values diverse perspectives and opposite views can stimulate innovation and lead significant advancements.

Additionally, embracing dissent requires acknowledging the public's role as consumers of scientific information. Misinformation can thrive in environments where scientific literacy is low. Therefore, enhancing public understanding through education is vital to ensure that dissent isn't perceived as a threat. Education programs that emphasize understanding scientific processes, how studies are conducted, and how evidence is evaluated can demystify the complexities that often cloud public discussions about scientific issues.

Moreover, policies themselves should recognize the importance of dissent by integrating transparent mechanisms that promote inclusion of diverse perspectives in scientific discourse. Creating transparent platforms for discussion can enable dissident voices to be heard without being prematurely silenced, while enhancing the integrity of scientific policymaking.

Consider alternative models like consensus conferences where stakeholders, including dissenters, come together to deliberate on contentious scientific topics with the aim of achieving mutual understanding. Such collaborative approaches can help clarify legitimate scientific disagreements from ideologically driven objections, thus enhancing the public's trust in science and policy.

Ultimately, the insistence on labeling medical dissent as dangerous necessitates re-evaluation. It requires examining not only the potential harms dissent might bring but also the harms of its suppression. The assumption that dissent inherently undermines public health must be replaced with recognition of its potential to inspire necessary and sometimes revolutionary innovations.

Scientific history is replete with instances where dissent against prevailing knowledge eventually led to significant advancements. From the rejection of bloodletting in favor of more effective medical practices to the acceptance of sanitation principles in disease prevention, progress has consistently depended on critically evaluating established norms through dissident lenses.

Therefore, it is imperative to rethink how dissent in medicine is perceived and responded to. By doing so, the medical community can better navigate the intricacies of scientific progress and public health, ensuring that valuable new insights aren't lost in the inertia of convention. Rather than perceiving dissent as anathema to science, embracing it as a vital component of the scientific method can enrich our collective understanding and lead to more robust and effective health practices.

## Concluding Thoughts

As we draw on the historical and contemporary examples of figures like Robert F. Kennedy Jr., it becomes clear that dissent in medicine is as much about shaping the future as it is about challenging the present. Exploring the rise in autism diagnoses post-COVID-19, opposition to mRNA vaccines, and the framing of dissent highlights how societal perceptions have long been contested territories. Now, more than ever, embracing a spectrum of viewpoints offers a chance not only to transform public health narratives but to empower individuals seeking truth and alternatives outside conventional frameworks. As we move forward, fostering open dialogue and inclusive discussions within the medical community could pave the way for innovations that challenge established norms while providing hope and alternative paths for those who feel overlooked by mainstream solutions. Understanding this dynamic prepares us for the forthcoming exploration into autism statistics and ongoing debates, where continuing the conversation with openness and curiosity becomes paramount in addressing complex health phenomena.

# Chapter 10 The Uncomfortable Truth About Medicine

Have you ever considered why our healthcare system seems more focused on managing diseases rather than curing them? For many, the promise of health care lies in finding solutions that restore us to full health. Yet, if you've ever found yourself or a loved one in a loop of continuous treatments and recurring doctor visits without any clear end in sight, you're not alone. Why is it that so many of us keep returning for the same treatments, clutching prescriptions that address symptoms but never seem to offer a definitive cure?

In this exploration of the medical industry, we'll delve into how financial incentives shape care decisions, prioritizing management over genuine healing. We will examine the systems at work that emphasize ongoing treatments instead of preventative measures or cures, considering the implications for patients who find themselves as perpetual subscribers to a model that doesn't favor their ultimate well-being. Through this chapter, we aim to uncover the underlying truths about these practices and explore what this means for those seeking real health solutions.

## Profiting from Disease Management

Let's dive into the complex relationship between medicine, profit, and patient care. Imagine a healthcare system where managing illness brings more revenue than curing it. For chronic disease management, this is often the case. Chronic diseases now account for about half of the healthcare expenditure, driven in part by management, rather than cure, of illness (Holman, 2020).

Consider how chronic illnesses, from diabetes to heart disease, require ongoing management. Rather than seeking cures, the healthcare system often emphasizes treatments that necessitate regular check-ups, medication adjustments, and specialist consultations. This model, often endorsed by the insurance systems and practitioners, maintains consistent revenue from patients who will need lifelong care. While it ensures immediate patient needs are covered, it rarely addresses the root causes of the diseases to offer sustainable solutions (Georgetown University, 2019).

In this context, financial incentives become a significant factor. Health plans, clinics, and physicians might find themselves pushed towards maintaining profitable chronic care routines over pursuing innovative cures that might not guarantee regular income streams. The model, while indeed facilitating comprehensive care, appears to create a paradox where reducing hospital visits and improving health do not always align with profit motives.

For instance, hospital incentives are often tied to the number of beds occupied, or the consistency of returning patients, as seen in traditional business models. More beds filled translates to more revenue, a model inherently conflicting with the notion of fewer patient visits due to effective cure strategies. The rise of chronic disease accounts for 44 percent of the population but demands a lion's share of healthcare expenditures (Georgetown University, 2019).

Moreover, managed care structures and financial compensation systems sometimes undermine drastic innovations in therapy that could otherwise remedy chronic conditions more effectively. The focus often lands on adjustments to financial frameworks such as managed care, pay-for-performance models, or shifting costs to patients through deductibles and copays, rather than fostering innovations in treatment options (Holman, 2020).

It's not just about sustaining profits, but about the mechanisms that allow profits to nationally and globally overshadow patient-centered care. Throughout the last few decades, despite advancements in technology and pharmacology, the financial weight has shifted towards managing and accommodating chronic conditions rather than heroic efforts to prevent their onset or resolve them completely.

For instance, while disease management programs prescribe medications and lifestyle adjustments that help maintain patients' health, they rarely align with innovations that promise outright cures, leaving healthcare systems focused on disease mitigation rather than eradication (Georgetown University, 2019).

Consider the story of Tom, a middle-aged man with diabetes. He regularly visits his doctor, fills prescriptions monthly, and attends diabetes management classes. Although these are essential practices to manage his condition and contribute to his quality of life, they also mean a recurring flow of income for healthcare providers. A strong support team, innovative treatments, and advanced diagnostic tools may exist, but they're embedded in a system where financial motivations favor maintenance over holistic exploration of cures.

Analyzing how we got here involves looking back at how healthcare evolved. Since the mid-20th century, emphasis gradually tilted towards managing long-term health conditions, sometimes at the cost of innovation in curative therapies. Insurance models, chronic disease coding, and benefit structures served their purpose but inadvertently established an economic reliance on disease management. They overshadow the significant efforts that could be made in areas like preventive care or therapeutic cures.

A deeper insight suggests the complexity goes beyond the hospital and into pharmaceutical companies and medical equipment manufacturers who thrive in the arena of recurring needs. Drug development, for example, sees a higher return on investment with medications designed for daily or ongoing consumption than for those ensuring one-time cures.

Recognizing this cycle prepares us to challenge it. Efforts towards change call for partnerships that promote breakthrough innovations alongside profit management in the healthcare arena. Advocacy for patient-first strategies emerges as paramount.

To drive reform requires realignment of incentives within the healthcare sector, prompting professionals to pioneer visionary therapies and accessible preventive care. This calls for a dynamic shift, one that leverages research, community health, and patient-centered approaches to dismantle enduring norms.

This reorientation provides a stepping stone into the following discussions around how pharmaceutical ties to regulatory bodies like the FDA shape these dynamics, further influencing the landscape of healthcare priorities. The ensuing exploration will delve into the intricate webs connecting pharmaceutical interests, federal oversight, and patient care expectations, aiming to unravel strategies for true patient empowerment and medical innovation.

# Interconnected Influence

In the world of pharmaceuticals, where managing disease often takes precedence over finding cures, a web of relationships between the FDA, Big Pharma, and global chemical companies tightly binds the industry. These connections influence not just the drugs that reach the market but also shape treatment protocols that lean more towards chronic management than curative solutions. This entanglement is a significant factor in maintaining the status quo, where pharmaceutical profitability overshadows patient welfare.

The ties between regulatory bodies and pharmaceutical giants are multi-layered and perplexing. Big Pharma's vast resources grant it unparalleled access to regulatory processes, often blurring the lines between government oversight and corporate influence. For instance, the FDA's role in scrutinizing drugs should ostensibly safeguard public health. Yet, these same organizations, like Big Pharma, are heavily involved in lobbying efforts that sway policies in their favor (Meller & Ahmed, 2019). This interconnection extends into the realm of active pharmaceutical ingredients (APIs), where a significant portion comes from overseas manufacturers. As of 2019, 72% of these manufacturing sites for the U.S. are outside the country, with 13% situated in China (Woodcock, 2019). The shift in production to countries with lower manufacturing costs presents challenges in maintaining quality control while creating a dependency on foreign supply chains.

As drug prices continue to soar, the interplay between Big Pharma and regulatory authorities becomes critical. The industry's revenue strategies often involve increasing medication costs disproportionately to inflation, a practice that has persisted despite administrative reassurances of reform (Meller & Ahmed, 2019). This relentless price hike neither correlates with innovative breakthroughs nor significant improvements in healthcare quality. It primarily reflects a profit-driven agenda, prioritizing consumption of medications over comprehensive healthcare solutions.

The relationship extends further into the realm of chemical companies, which supply essential raw materials for pharmaceutical production. The global nature of these supply chains means that cost-reduction strategies, such as outsourcing, frequently undermine both environmental and ethical standards.

The Chinese production boom in APIs is partly due to lower operational costs, including lenient environmental regulations (Woodcock, 2019). While these practices trim costs for companies, they contribute to pollution and health risks in production countries, with ripple effects felt globally.

The influence of these companies often steers the direction of drug research and availability. Significant financial stakes in maintaining long-term medication regimens divert attention from potentially disruptive cures or innovations. The FDA's partnership with these entities can sometimes appear complicit in maintaining treatment paradigms rather than endorsing transformative cures. Corporate interests frequently guide the approval processes, ensuring that financially beneficial drugs get greenlighted while sidelining less profitable but potentially curative research paths.

Concrete examples abound in examining how corporate interests intertwine with regulatory decisions. The recall of contaminated or ineffective medications occurs amidst complex negotiations that occasionally favor corporate damage control over immediate public health responses. The extended time it can take for these issues to be rectified highlights a regulatory sluggishness exacerbated by industrial influence (Woodcock, 2019). The intricate dance between profit-making and patient safety seesaws precariously, often tipping towards industrial interests.

Consider, for example, the contentious practices around drug patents and the evergreen strategies employed by pharmaceutical companies to extend their market monopolies. Such tactics underscore a broader effort to prolong profit cycles rather than expediting the advent of generic, cost-effective alternatives that could radically reduce healthcare expenses for patients. This interplay between industry innovation and regulatory approval requires vigilant scrutiny to safeguard against exploitation (Meller & Ahmed, 2019).

It's crucial to understand the ramifications for patient outcomes. The prioritization of treatment over cure means many diseases remain chronic on purpose. While steady demand ensures reliable revenue streams for companies, patients face continuously climbing expenses and prolonged health challenges. Exploring the drugs and treatments the FDA approves reveals a pattern: chronic condition management continues unperturbed, whereas fewer dollars funnel into research for cures that might upend this equilibrium.

Transiting smoothly to the next section of the chapter, it's vital to recognize the historical challenges posed by influential pharmaceutical players like Bayer. Their lasting imprint on the pharmaceutical-industrial complex provides a lens through which contemporary issues can be better understood. The legacy of companies like Bayer showcases how intricate the dance between innovation, regulatory oversight, and corporate interest has always been. From their foundation to their current stature, these entities have shaped and defined much of the modern medical landscape.

The historical context, particularly around Bayer and its pivotal role in establishing many of the norms in the pharmaceutical industry, continues to reverberate today. It is a legacy marked by both innovation and controversy, reflective of ambitious goals often clashing with ethical considerations. Understanding their past advancements and strategic moves offers a rich tapestry of lessons and cautions.

Thus, examining the pivotal roles played by these intersecting forces suggests a complex lattice of influence and agenda-setting that is as much about economic interests as it is about healthcare imperatives. As we look to the next part of this exploration, where we delve deeper into the legacy of global players like Bayer, it becomes crucial to continue dissecting these legacy influences to discern their contemporary implications on patient care and the pursuit of innovation in medicine.

# Historical Industrial Complex

Picking up from the intricate ties between regulatory agencies, Big Pharma, and global chemical companies, the story pivots towards Bayer, a prime historical specimen of the pharmaceutical-industrial complex. A brand synonymous with both innovation and controversy, Bayer's trajectory exemplifies how past alliances continue to shape medicine today. From its early days, Bayer carved a name in the industry. The company revolutionized medicine in the 19th century by introducing Aspirin, embedding itself into healthcare. However, it wasn't just their products that left a mark. Their intertwining with the industry's fabric began a pattern of prioritizing disease management over cures, a trend still prevalent.

Bayer's initiatives, particularly in antibiotics, are case studies of commercial interest intersecting with healthcare priorities. Notoriously, Bayer saw success in antibiotics with the introduction of Cipro during the late 1980s (Skender, 2024). The rise of antibiotic-resistant strains presented an opportunity for profits, yet Bayer's decisions reflected the commercial weight over therapeutic advancements. Rather than exploring radically new compounds, the company leveraged existing markets, aligning with Akan Bezsonkov's insights of profit dictating research paths. The economic imperatives often meant sidelining non-lucrative disease areas, suggesting a disquieting alignment of market incentives over patient outcomes (Mintz, 2011).

Symbolically, Bayer's memorial for forced laborers in Leverkusen stands as a poignant reminder of an era driven by an aggressive industrially dominated ethos (History, 2021). It reflects the historical complexities where progress was sometimes drug along with ethical compromises. By acknowledging its past, Bayer implicitly points to the deep interconnectedness of socio-political dynamics with corporate evolution, furthering the narrative of prioritizing systemic management over innovation in healing.

Despite its potent role in antibiotics, with seminal discoveries, Bayer struggled in maintaining competitiveness due to growing industry demands and regulatory complexities (Achilladelis and Antonakis, 2001). The transition away from antibiotic innovations to more lucrative markets like oncology exemplifies a strategic pivot seen across Big Pharma, where financial returns took precedence over continuing advances in critical therapeutic areas. This withdrawal also highlighted how even successful entities like Bayer can succumb to the industrial pressure, stymieing potentially groundbreaking treatments (Mintz, 2011; Skender, 2024).

The company's extensive partnership with academic and medical institutions drove significant advancements, presenting a dual-edged sword. On one side, it spurred innovation, pooling intellectual resources for new medical breakthroughs. Yet, it inherently tied academic pursuits with commercial objectives, emphasizing market demand-fueled competition over fundamental cures (Verg, 1988). The commercial frameworks built around resistance, growth expectations, and stricter regulations further choked the momentum, indicating an intricate entanglement not easily undone by traditional talent alone.

This section serves to unveil Bayer as a symptom and a driver of a paradigm where management often overshadows cures. It illustrates how historical players laid the groundwork for current systemic tendencies, focusing more on alleviating symptoms than eradicating illnesses. The ethos that managed to persist is woven into the consciousness of today's medical landscape, where drug resistance battles are fought as much in boardrooms as in laboratories.

Exploring specific incidents deepens this understanding further. For instance, Bayer engineers involved in research during the antibiotic heyday essentially crafted processes boosting drug yields rather than pioneering completely new classes (Dalhoff, 2008a). While patenting posed a regulatory labyrinth, conserving shareholder value sometimes overshadowed the ethical imperative to innovate. This mirrors a broader industrial tendency to hedge innovations against profitable safety nets, ensuring market stability over disruptive discoveries (Gradmann, 2016).

Moreover, Bayer's institution of forums like the "Innovation Perspective '97" underscores its narrative control within the industry, framing itself as both a benefactor and benefactor-in-chief (Verg, 1988). By invoking Schumpeter's notion of entrepreneurship and innovation, the company synchronized its brand identity with capitalist ideals, reinforcing an entrenched business-centric approach to healthcare — management over cure, packaged in ingenuity.

Each point made exemplifies a broader theme of system-oriented behavior over patient-centered care. Bayer's story, thus, is not redundant but emergent within this narrative of interwoven interests, serving as a chisel, carving commercial imperatives into healthcare's bedrock. The industry's profit-oriented nature exacerbated this pattern, repeatedly tilting balance towards economic outcomes rather than anchoring patient welfare with breakthroughs.

Concluding this section, the next explores why patient compliance seems pre-programmed into the medical systems themselves. Bayer's framework shifts our focus towards what the coming content will expound: the hierarchical dynamics compelling patients to obey rather than challenge industrial dictates. The sinuous path from evident Bayer strategies to systemic patient control will transition into examining Clark's perspective — detoxification as an elemental healing method. This shift will unveil how historical industry dominions direct present patient interactions, crafting a narrative exploring compliance amid contested health paradigms.

# Patient Compliance vs. Autonomy

The close historical connection between Bayer and the broader pharmaceutical-industrial complex reveals how past partnerships shape today's medical practices. These enduring ties illustrate a focus on treatment, often at the expense of thorough cures, due to underlying industry interests. These historical roots manifest in a system that often encourages unquestioning adherence rather than encouraging critical thought among patients. This inclination is evident as patients are often conditioned to comply with medical authorities, trusting branded medications and figures, and showing compliance towards their recommendations without probing the deeper implications. This dynamic persists because the system often prioritizes disease management while viewing genuine cures as disruptive to ongoing medical revenue streams.

At the heart of this medical obedience lies an educational narrative that consistently emphasizes the authority of medical professionals. From early encounters with doctors, patients learn to regard medical advice as irrefutable. Institutional structures reinforce this dynamic, relying on compliance to streamline treatment protocols and achieve uniform results. Patients following this path of least resistance accept prescriptions and treatments without considering why these treatments are prescribed in the first place. This approach aligns with financial motivations within the medical industry that benefit from repeat patients and continuous treatment cycles.

Hulda Clark offers a counter-narrative through her emphasis on detoxification and toxin removal. Clark argues that self-healing emerges when the body is free from the overwhelming interference of external substances. According to her perspective, chronic conditions stem not from inherent deficiencies but from the accumulated effects of pollutants, chemicals, and waste that burden the body. Thus, by eliminating these toxins, the body can restore its natural equilibrium and trigger healing processes. This approach starkly contrasts with mainstream practices that often seek quick fixes through pharmaceuticals, which sometimes introduce additional substances to the body instead of eliminating them.

Concrete examples illustrate how patients are led to accept and comply with medical advice without question. Case studies reveal individuals pursuing aggressive treatment regimens for chronic conditions without exploring alternative solutions. These patients too often succumb to the pressure of adhering to a regimen that validates the medical system's expertise while leaving little room to interrogate the merits of such treatments. This pattern engrains a behavior that devalues personal agency and the exploration of self-healing methods. However, those who challenge this norm often encounter skepticism from both medical professionals and acquaintances who place their beliefs in more widely accepted practices.

Clark's philosophy of detoxification posits that the body can initiate its natural recovery mechanisms when given the opportunity. By eliminating harmful substances from their lifestyle, patients can potentially reevaluate their health. Testimonials from those adopting detoxification methods share stories of relief from chronic pain, improvement in energy levels, and renewed mental clarity. These narratives are compelling as they highlight shifts in health that mainstream treatments had marginally impacted.

For example, individuals suffering from migraines often find conventional medications offer only temporary relief, pushing them into a cycle of dependency. In contrast, some who embrace detoxification regimens report long-lasting improvement without ongoing medication. Through diet changes, elimination of processed foods, and focus on organic ingredients, some patients observe remarkable transformations, suggesting efficacy in Clark's methods. Their stories challenge the equilibrium of the accepted medical wisdom which can overly rely on pharmaceuticals.

By emphasizing her perspective, Clark draws attention to a fundamental shift in patient behavior. Rather than obediently following prescribed treatment paths, patients regain control over their health through informed choice. These insights reveal a gap between current medical practices and the potential for self-healing. They underscore a recurring issue where the deterrence of critical engagement limits possibilities for innovative health approaches.

To realign the medical industry towards empowering patients, there is a need for structural change. This shift requires re-evaluating the symbiotic relationship between pharmaceutical companies and regulatory bodies to ensure that genuine innovation in self-healing, rather than simply perpetuating cycles of treatment, becomes an industry focus. Recognizing patients as active participants in their care rather than passive recipients allows for a more nuanced understanding of health.

The medical field's inclination towards patient compliance stems from deep historical ties and economic interests. Patients cultivated in this system often face discouragement when posing questions about their treatment plans. However, by exploring alternative modalities like Clark's toxin removal, opportunities for personal empowerment and self-recovery surface. Her philosophy represents a shift from the traditional path, urging an examination of inherent possibilities within the human body for renewal and healing. It advocates an important dialogue concerning the balance between established medical practices and emerging self-reliant approaches to health.

# Final Thoughts

**The exploration of how the medical industry prioritizes management over cures reveals a system driven by profit rather than patient well-being. The broader implications for patients include an entrenched cycle where chronic conditions are managed for sustained revenue, often at the expense of innovative curative efforts. By understanding this dynamic, there's potential to rethink healthcare incentives. Now that we recognize the systemic focus on treatment rather than prevention or cure, we can advocate for a shift towards truly patient-centered care. This involves partnering with forward-thinking practitioners and championing approaches that prioritize genuine healing. The insights gained compel us to challenge existing paradigms and embrace treatments that empower individuals and reduce dependency on lifelong disease management.**

# Chapter 11 A Legacy They Couldn't Kill

Imagine a world where your health choices are dictated not by what you believe is best for your body, but by external forces silencing alternative voices. This was the reality faced by a groundbreaking figure in health and wellness, whose innovative ideas were met with relentless efforts to suppress them. Yet, her legacy persisted. From her popular books that found their way into eager hands despite attempts at censorship, to her Zapper device sought by those exploring holistic solutions, every effort to quash her influence only fueled greater curiosity and demand.

In communities across digital landscapes, her teachings have not only survived but thrived, illustrating how resilient and necessary her contributions are to health discourse. Her work serves as a beacon for those seeking alternatives outside conventional medicine—those who refuse to be boxed into mainstream narratives, who value self-healing and medical freedom. As we dive into this chapter, we'll explore the tenacity of her legacy, unraveling how her pioneering ideas continue to challenge and inspire amidst ongoing cultural resistance.

## Despite silencing, her books still sell. People still search for her Zapper.

Despite attempts to suppress her work, the legacy of our pioneering figure in health and wellness thrives. Her ideas remain vibrant and inspiring, which is evident when discussing her popular books and sought-after Zapper. The story here isn't so much about overcoming censorship but the resilience and necessity of her contributions to discussions on health alternatives. In inaccessible settings, from school libraries to general community access points, book bans have only intensified attention on controversial works. Authors like Kyle Lukoff and others, covered by CNN's report, have faced profound challenges with their works being banned yet still maintain an ability to connect with readers (Andrew, 2023). This cultural resistance against thought suppression parallels the ongoing demand for our subject's work, despite attempts to shut it down.

Book bans and soft censorship illuminate a broader trend of restricting access to diverse ideas and materials. In the same vein, an alarming increase in book behaviors signals a broader movement seeking to silence diverse voices and viewpoints (Meehan, 2024). These initiatives often claim to protect but instead stifle creativity and self-expression. Similar to Kyle Lukoff's experience, where recognition due to controversy didn't translate into increased sales, our innovator's work didn't vanish under pressure. Her books, having been shared through formal and informal networks, hold spaces within the health and wellness community. They continue to be a source of knowledge and exploration for those seeking alternatives. An insightful comment from Laurie Halse Anderson encapsulates this perspective — writing for young people demands attentiveness to their challenges and offers stories they identify with. Her point reinforces the notion that the demand for diverse narratives echoes the enduring relevance of our subject's unique contributions (Meehan, 2024).

In the narratives of suppressed authors, substantial parallels emerge that resonate with her work still living on in public consciousness. Authors have faced censorial climates focusing heavily on sexual and racial content, much of it clearly reflected in analyses conducted by entities like PEN America (Meehan, 2024). These actions have not succeeded in extinguishing the public's interest. It's a testament to the appeal that when readers become aware of the suppression of ideas, those works often garner a cult following; they represent the embodiment of ideas that should not be silenced. Our health and wellness figure represents a cornerstone in this dialogue, her books serving not only as texts but as symbols of resistance against conformity and standardization in health narratives.

Such continuing demand is conspicuously illuminated by the search for her Zapper, akin to the sought-after themes and messages in books that challenge prevailing norms. The Zapper represents more than just a device; it's become an icon of her philosophy and her enduring influence. A reliable indicator of her impact, the consistent interest in acquiring her Zapper proves instrumental in highlighting how an entrenched audience continues to explore and engage with her ideas, nurturing the legacy of her innovations in alternative health. This search for knowledge signals a wider curiosity about integrating diverse wellness practices into mainstream health approaches.

Testimonies from those exploring alternative health solutions underscore how her inventions open dialogues about healing and wellness. The Zapper, in this sense, has shifted from a niche interest into a central piece of conversation around holistic health. The persistence in seeking it even now reflects a broader audience willing to dig deeper for health narratives and solutions that resonate on a personal level.

As health discourse evolves, echoing back to 2023's narrative on book bans highlights how controversies inadvertently boost public curiosity. Readers and consumers, often driven by narratives around censorship, become more inclined to seek out forbidden works or tools, simply fueled by the intrigue and validation from others who felt similarly. This interconnectedness in seeking meaningful interactions with content mirrors the sustained interest in our figure's works.

Moreover, seeing how banned authors have had their followings increase online and offline creates a fascinating parallel with how our innovator's videos are currently finding a home on YouTube and alternative platforms. In the transition, books and devices like the Zapper pivot into communities where their messages are preserved and propagated, using newer forms of media. Viewers take to these platforms to document, discuss, and advise on using such alternative perspectives, ensuring the continuum of these ideas beyond what traditional censorship might hinder.

By speaking directly to our pioneer's tenacity in facing down significant cultural and institutional barriers, we acknowledge her tremendous influence across mediums. Her work remains indispensable as it broadens the possibilities of self-care narratives. The digital landscape has become fertile ground for her ideas to circulate freely, demonstrating how once niche interests now penetrate mainstream consciousness and hint at larger shifts in public health discourse.

The ensuing section we transition to delves into how her videos continue to captivate audiences on YouTube and parallel platforms, naturally extending from the well-established popularity of her books and the Zapper searches. By tapping into this digital transformation, her ideas reach new demographic groups, connecting people with diverse interests and igniting conversations about holistic health. This evolution illustrates a compelling narrative about the unstoppable spread of ideas that, despite attempts at suppression, continue thriving in ever-more inventive ways. It's about maintaining momentum, ensuring that even if books and gadgets face hurdles, the outreach of this trailblazer's legacy adapts fluidly to the conditions.

# Her videos circulate on YouTube and alternative platforms.

In the world of alternative health, the legacy of this wellness pioneer continues to shine brightly. Online communities have taken up the torch, sharing insights and amplifying the teachings that have transcended her physical books and sought-after devices, like the Zapper. Her influence finds new life in the digital realm, far from the pages of her beloved tomes or the physical products that once filled countless orders.

On forums such as Reddit's r/holistichealth, discussions thrive about the practical applications of her protocols, creating an ever-evolving tapestry of collective knowledge. Users eagerly exchange success stories, troubleshoot issues, and provide support, all of which turns these digital spaces into living extensions of her teachings. Telegram channels, known for their encrypted messaging and community features, host vibrant discussions where members not only share experiences but also collaborate on ways to improve and tailor protocols to fit their individual needs. These platforms foster environments where individuals feel safe and empowered to explore alternative health solutions without fear of judgment or reprisal.

Specific YouTube channels dedicated to holistic wellness showcase content inspired by her methods, often featuring testimonials from those who credit her protocols with significant improvements in their health. Videos demonstrating 'Zapper' usage highlight enthusiastic community members eager to share their firsthand experiences. This visual medium serves as an accessible starting point for newcomers while offering seasoned followers an opportunity to refine their understanding and implementation of the techniques. Comments sections become hotspots for information exchange, question-and-answer sessions, and even encouragement among viewers.

Inside private Facebook groups, detailed anecdotes and success stories recalculate belief even from skeptical corners. Members discuss dietary changes, detoxification protocols, and lifestyle modifications that align with her teachings, delivering proof that interest in her methods hasn't diminished over time. This constant interaction and feedback loop builds a layer of trust within these communities, reinforcing her protocols as viable alternatives to conventional medicine.

Continual interest in her work has fueled the birth of an overarching DIY health movement. A growing number of people have taken her concepts of self-testing and self-healing to heart, extending the reach of her advice into realms like personalized health monitoring and the use of wearable technology. This movement champions the idea that individuals can take charge of their health through mindfulness, informed choices, and community support. The principles of self-responsibility promoted by these communities embody her vision of a future where personal health management becomes a collaborative, rather than prescriptive, endeavor.

Concrete examples abound, exemplifying how community members draw strength and empowerment from their shared journeys. In one notable case, a digital marketing strategist who was initially skeptical about holistic protocols embraced her teachings after joining a community that collectively celebrated small victories and addressed setbacks with empathy and understanding. This newfound confidence allowed her to explore additional avenues of personal health improvements, cementing her belief in this alternative path to wellness.

Another inspiring story involves a retired teacher who discovered that simple dietary adjustments recommended by the community had profound effects on her chronic ailments. Her testimonial, shared on multiple platforms, inspired countless others to take the plunge, contributing to an ever-increasing repository of endorsements that breathed new life into the protocols.

As community members conquer personal health challenges, they contribute their findings back to the groups—each achievement recorded as a testament to her enduring influence. This cyclical exchange keeps interest alight and allows the teachings to remain relevant today, unshackling them from the static nature of print and empowering them in the mutable space of online discourse.

These communities don't exist in isolation. They often overlap with larger digital ecosystems that further inspire and refine personal health innovations. Cross-platform discussions involve everything from insights on integrating digital tools into wellness plans to philosophical debates on the future of health in the age of information. Members cherish the adaptability of online spaces, where collaborative learning steps to the forefront, crafting a new kind of pedagogy that remains faithful to her pioneering vision.

Turning toward the future, discussions increasingly anticipate the rise of technologies like biofeedback devices and health-tracking apps, empowered by a foundation rooted in her teachings. Community-driven DIY health kits, developed based on shared protocols, hint at an emerging market where innovation meets practicality. These tools guide enthusiasts through the myriad steps of self-care, marrying modern technology with age-old wisdom.

As this section bridges to those that follow, the discussion will naturally segue into the intersections of traditional and modern methods, mapping out how her teachings inspire ongoing innovation. The increased attention on self-testing, holistic diagnostics, and individual accountability represents a logical evolution of her life's work—one that online communities perpetually nurture and champion.

Through every social media post, online conversation, and shared success, the principles she introduced are redefined and reexamined, ensuring her legacy remains not merely alive but in full bloom. The grassroots movement she sparked through her protocols and teachings illuminates a path for those drawn to holistic health, encouraging them to step away from the well-trodden trail and onto a journey of discovery that's deeply personal and profoundly communal.

## Online communities still follow her protocols and share results.

Previously, we explored how her videos circulate on platforms like YouTube, establishing a dynamic environment where her teachings perpetuate and gather momentum. This digital ecosystem plays a crucial role in shaping the vibrant communities devoted to practicing and sharing experiences grounded in her protocols. Online platforms not only amplify her influence but serve as the cornerstone for communities that passionately adhere to her methods, fostering a collective that both preserves and propels her legacy. By focusing on these digital networks, we see how individuals globally remain engaged in conversations that honor and expand upon her original insights.

Online communities emerge as essential arteries in the digital landscape, channeling the lifeblood of her teachings and supporting a vast array of health enthusiasts who gather to share their journeys. These groups act as vibrant spaces where community members relay personal narratives, support one another, and offer advice and encouragement. The testimonials shared within these circles often highlight transformative results, showcasing how users of her protocols report improvements in health and well-being. Sharing testimonials and outcomes in these arenas offers both validation and motivation, reinforcing commitment to her teachings. This sharing not only deepens personal engagement but also invites curious onlookers to explore these wellness avenues.

The dedication seen in these online groups demonstrates the profound impact her teachings have forged across diverse communities. Participants often regard themselves as caretakers of a legacy, tasked with transmitting and sustaining her protocols. They leverage digital tools to document triumphs and setbacks, troubleshoot challenges, and beta-test new insights that might emerge within the boundaries of her original teachings. Frequently, forums highlight specific health strategies, detailing methods or adaptations employed by members to suit varying personal circumstances. Such exchanges cultivate a rich tapestry of experiences, collectively reinforcing the enduring relevance of her work to new and seasoned adherents alike.

The practices these communities engage in can be detailed and impactful. For instance, members regularly exchange information about dietary protocols, compare notes on ingredient sourcing, and troubleshoot the nuances of dietary interventions. In many forums, individuals post detailed accounts of their journeys, from the initial adoption of her methods to the ongoing tweaks that optimize their outcomes. This type of peer-reviewed self-diagnosis serves as a powerful tool, offering both a sense of community and a platform for practical knowledge exchange. Among the most valuable aspects of these interactions is the reassurance members provide to those encountering difficulties, fostering a culture that thrives on mutual aid and continuous improvement.

Moreover, the impact of these online communities extends beyond anecdotal sharing. Many groups encourage members to engage in citizen science, participating in personal experiments that document efficacy and contribute to collective knowledge. Whether it's monitoring health markers or utilizing apps to track behavioral changes, these community-driven efforts provide valuable insights into the effectiveness of her protocols in real-world settings. Through shared spreadsheets, journals, and detailed accounts, these digital assemblies function as informal research collaboratives, charting new territories that traditional science may yet to explore or validate.

The collective wisdom emanating from these discussions not only provides a blueprint for personal health endeavors but also inspires broader shifts towards proactive health management. By participating in these communities, many individuals develop a robust understanding of self-care practices that empower them to manage their wellness independently. This transition to self-directed health echoes the sentiments of a DIY health movement inspired by her teachings, fostering a landscape where individuals are encouraged to deepen their understanding of how lifestyle choices influence their well-being.

The fervor demonstrated in online discussions underscores the active participation and profound commitment members bring to these forums. Navigating various digital spaces, participants form tight-knit communities where knowledge exchange becomes the keystroke currency that enriches everyone involved. This model of learning and sharing has a compounding effect, attracting new members who eagerly delve into a trove of grassroots insights, further expanding the community and reinforcing this ever-growing cycle of collective growth and discovery.

Ultimately, these online ecosystems function as vibrant, living archives of her health and wellness teachings, preserving their relevance and accessibility. The diligent engagement of members ensures continual re-evaluation and innovation within her prescribed frameworks, reflecting evolving perspectives and new wellness challenges. At its core, the dynamic nature of these digital collectives ensures that her legacy remains not only a testament to past meritorious practices but a thriving, adaptable paradigm of holistic health management suited for modern times.

As we transition to exploring the DIY health movement catalyzed by her philosophies, it's evident how these online communities represent the genesis of self-testing, self-healing, and self-responsibility paradigms. Rooted in shared experiences and communal learning, participants are empowered to craft individualized health trajectories that embody personal agency and accountability. The collective efforts within these digital gatherings highlight a widespread embrace of self-directed wellness approaches, underscoring how collaboration and shared knowledge inspire individuals to take charge of their health journeys. Through this communal enterprise, her legacy not only perseveres but actively evolves, inviting ever-more individuals to partake in and enrich the shared mission of holistic harmony and healthful living.

# DIY health movement inspired by Clark—self-testing, self-healing, self-responsibility.

The digital age has transformed how we approach health, offering new platforms to exchange tips, share stories, and reinforce community bonds. The online communities, once considered niche gatherings, now act as robust ecosystems nurturing alternative health ideas. This newfound connectivity plays a crucial role in sustaining the teachings of our featured health advocate. Members of these communities consistently adapt and implement her protocols, demonstrating the enduring strength and relevance of her guidance. From here, the transition to the wider DIY health movement, born from her influence, is seamless.

In the DIY health movement, self-testing has emerged as a testament to the faith people place in their ability to understand and take control of their health. Rather than seeing health as a black box understood only by professionals, her philosophy posits that individuals can learn to analyze their body's signals and respond accordingly. For example, many have turned to home testing kits to monitor conditions like vitamin deficiencies or hormone levels. By using these kits, individuals not only gain insights into their internal health landscape but also cultivate a form of self-awareness that empowers them to make informed health decisions.

This growing empowerment sees people using alternative methods, like herbal remedies and dietary adjustments, as forms of self-healing. The core idea here isn't just self-medication; it's about fostering a deeper connection with one's body and understanding its unique needs. Consider those who have adopted her suggestions for managing stress through meditation and mindfulness. These practices of self-healing emphasize the role of mental well-being, aligning with broader research that highlights how psychological health influences physical health outcomes (Martinez et al., 2021).

The commitment to self-responsibility she advocates pushes people to question conventional health pathways. Her teaching inspires them to venture beyond traditional medicine, seeking solutions that integrate rather than segregate personal health accountability and professional advice. In practice, this manifests as a balanced partnership with healthcare providers, a sentiment echoed in the literature emphasizing shared decision-making between patients and physicians (Paterick et al., 2017). By consciously deciding to take responsibility, not only do people feel more in control, but they also often experience improved health outcomes as active participants in their wellness journey.

The indispensability of patient education, as supported by self-care research, underpins this movement. Educating oneself about one's condition eradicates helplessness, lifting the individual above passive acceptance. Her teachings align with the view that improving health literacy leads to better adherence to positive lifestyle changes like diet and exercise, ultimately reducing risks associated with chronic diseases (Martinez et al., 2021).

This ownership over health brings a sense of community reflection, where one's journey motivates others to embark on their paths. We see individuals sharing personal triumphs over lifestyle diseases such as hypertension or diabetes, motivated by their adherence to her holistic lifestyle suggestions. Sharing success stories fosters solidarity and hope amongst those struggling with similar conditions, proving that her legacy is indeed alive and continues to offer an alternative route to health.

Her influence extends to resistance against misinformation that often accompanies mainstream narratives. This resistance is not merely adversarial but serves as a reminder that different perspectives not only deserve attention but warrant exploration. This attitude empowers individuals to face medical proposals or diagnoses with informed skepticism, questioning and validating the information through multiple sources, thus fostering an environment of informed consent and autonomy.

Even amidst opposition from some sectors eager to dismiss these methods, her followers persist, driven by practical success and personal transformations. For instance, anecdotes abound of individuals supplementing conventional treatments with alternative practices, reporting perceived increases in efficacy and satisfaction. These testimonies align with the principles of informed medical choice, where decisions are collaborative, respecting patient autonomy in the healthcare process (Paterick et al., 2017).

The idea of self-care, once confined within narrow definitions, now flourishes broadly thanks to the path she charted. Exploring one's path to health through awareness, self-control, and self-reliance strengthens the individual's role in the healthcare dialogue. The multilayered concept of self-care suggests that despite the escalation of chronic diseases, individuals harness the power to impact their health destinies positively (Martinez et al., 2021).

As the DIY health movement continues to evolve, the tenets laid down by our health advocate remind us that health is not a one-size-fits-all discipline. Her teachings encourage embracing a personalized approach, integrating personal preference and professional guidance into a cohesive health strategy. This personalization stands against the uniformity in treatments often promoted in institutional healthcare, emphasizing that individuality matters significantly in health and wellness outcomes.

The narrative she fosters challenges the validity of conventional healthcare as the sole authority on wellness. Instead, her influence encourages a symbiotic relationship, where alternative practices contribute meaningfully to overall health strategies. Such integration not only validates her legacy but underscores how deeply her teachings resonate with those battling chronic illnesses or seeking truth in their health journeys.

By continually engaging with her philosophy and adapting it into modern contexts, individuals across the globe reaffirm the broad appeal and efficacy of these methods. Transforming health care from a passive act to an active collaboration marks a powerful shift towards empowerment. This shift doesn't undermine conventional medicine; instead, it invigorates the healthcare landscape to embrace diverse practices, echoing the very essence of her teachings that have carved an unerasable path in today's health scene.

## The Clark Protocol lives on, underground—but alive.

The Tijuana clinic Dr. Clark founded is no longer in operation following her passing in 2009. While her methods and legacy continue to be discussed online, the physical clinic no longer exists.

Despite efforts to suppress her pioneering work in health and wellness, the legacy of this trailblazer persists, driven by an unwavering community seeking genuine alternatives. The digital age has become a bastion for her teachings, amplifying them across platforms like YouTube and Telegram, where enthusiastic followers exchange insights and experiences. Her influence endures through a robust dialogue on holistic approaches, inspiring a global do-it-yourself health movement that prioritizes self-awareness and informed choices over passive acceptance. Empowered individuals now explore home-testing kits and mindful practices, embracing their unique health journeys while challenging mainstream narratives. As her ideas intertwine with modern health dialogues, they continue to reshape perceptions and inspire resilience against conformity. In recognizing the power within these alternative communities, we understand that her contributions are more vital than ever, charting a path not only towards individual well-being but also collective empowerment. Now that these alternative solutions have gained traction, there's potential for broader transformation in how people view and manage personal health, blending holistic and conventional wisdom for a healthier future.

# Chapter 12 What They Don't Want You to Know

Do you remember as a child being told to eat your fruits and vegetables because they're good for you? Imagine if every apple, carrot, or piece of lettuce was carrying more than just vitamins and minerals. Sarah, a young mother striving to give her family the healthiest meals possible, never suspected these wholesome foods could harbor hidden dangers. After all, they looked fresh and nutritious, just like those on any grocery store shelf. It wasn't until her son experienced mysterious stomach pains that lasted weeks, despite a diet rich in fresh produce, that she began to question what these foods might truly contain. Her search led her down an unexpected path, revealing unsettling truths buried beneath the vibrant surfaces of everyday foods.

The reality is, our daily diets may not be as safe as we believe. Many of us trust that the items filling our shopping carts are regulated and checked, but lurking within our food supply are unseen threats that can impact our health over time. In this chapter, we'll delve into the world of food contaminants—from parasites and toxins to dyes and heavy metals—exposing how these elements make their way onto our dinner plates.

# Dangers of Our Food Supply

Every time you eat simple foods like fruits and vegetables, you're potentially ingesting more than nutrition. Parasites such as tapeworms and roundworms become unintended guests in our foods. While not all parasites lurk in your salad bowl, inadequate cleaning exposes you to these critters that can lead to gastrointestinal issues, muscle pain, and a compromised immune system. For example, undercooked pork may contain larvae of the Trichinella parasite, a notorious source of discomfort.

Consider mycotoxins, a group of naturally-occurring toxins produced by fungi found primarily in grains and nuts. Take aflatoxins, for example, which commonly contaminate peanuts and maize. Chronic exposure to aflatoxins contributes significantly to liver cancer, as illustrated by alarming studies in particular parts of Africa and Asia. Even low-level exposure over time risks compromising liver function, leading to severe health repercussions. The impact aligns with findings linking chemical contaminants to chronic intestinal inflammation seen in colitis models (Liu et al., 2025).

Meanwhile, azo dyes are synthetic colorants widely used to improve the appearance of foods. Used to brighten visually dull groceries, they sneak into our lives masked as harmless additives. But studies show the potential of azo dyes to induce allergic reactions or even stir hyperactivity in children. In particular, tartrazine, found in candies and sodas, is notorious for causing urticaria and asthma symptoms. These colorants, though seemingly benign, act like slow catalysts for ongoing health battles without the uptick of their behind-the-scenes consequences.

Similarly, heavy metals worm their way into food through various channels like soil contamination and industrial pollution. Metals such as cadmium, lead, and mercury find their path into our diets through rice, fish, broccoli, and more. Mercury levels in fish like swordfish can lead to neurological abnormalities, a hazard especially prevalent in pregnant women and children due to developmental risks. Frequent lead exposure prompts behavioral and cognitive issues, with links pointing towards pervasive microplastic contamination in ecosystems and food chains (Walraven et al., 2024).

While each of these elements alone poses its challenges, their cumulative presence in daily diets creates a cocktail of hazards that raise health concerns globally. The invisible and pervasive nature of these contaminants accents how consumption opens doors to various invisible threats. This resonance becomes apparent when considering pesticide residues, such as organochlorine, notably impacting conditions like Inflammatory Bowel Disease (IBD) (Walraven et al., 2024). The pesticides remain in the atmosphere even after numerous bans, inevitably trickling their way into food chains and raising substantial human health implications.

The transformative nature of modern agriculture contributes immeasurably to these risks. They navigate and settle quietly within crops as widespread pesticide use effectively deteriorates soil integrity over time. Chemical and biological dynamics hence interplay, escalating from cellular to ecological levels unpredictably. Recent strides in agricultural nanostructure applications work toward identifying food contaminants more effectively, signaling potential mitigation measures against these harmful residues (Liu et al., 2025).

Persistent pesticide residue challenges become complicated not only as isolated threats but also via the synthetic chemical interactions they participate in within the human biome. Even within the intestinal environment, disrupted microbiome balance aligns with largescale ingestion repercussions woven into suppressed immune response symptoms (Walraven et al., 2024). The prolific emergence of such synthetic infiltrations begs for conscious scrutiny toward self-sustainability approaches, engendering alternative food practices over high dependency energy-dense consumables.

The chemical contamination doesn't stop at what we choose to consume. Food packaging materials often perpetuate these additives, leaching more synthetic particles into our food. These practices blur the lines between internal consumption choices and external environmental influences, fostering pronounced cascading health effects. It's as if we're being breached at every corner by an overwhelming flow of synthetic incursion, beyond what is readily monitored and tracked.

There is a compelling need for consumers to push boundaries in active decision-making, adopting awareness over convenience. Family choices spanning prebiotic support and stringent local produce sourcing showcase the efficacy of organic refinement. Further consumer-driven advocacy on transparent labeling battles creates tentative deterrents to widespread hidden chemical proliferation within food supplies.

The narratives around parasite, mycotoxin, azo dye, and heavy metal prevalence reveal deep-rooted contamination stakes across the food spectrum. Repeated exposure to the cumulative low dosages of such elements seeds long-term physical imbalances. Consumer consciousness pushes for transparency, calling for improved systemic and nutritional practices. Glimpses of hope surface, reflective of informed behavioral choices and policy advocacy leveraging awareness as potent amplifiers for change.

The narrative urgency ties smoothly to a revelation of carcinogenic compounds lurking in common personal grooming products. Armed with systemic risk knowledge, you can transition towards unpacking these common but lesser heeded risks present in toothpaste, hair dye, and shampoo. The path to mindful consumerism involves demystifying and replacing petrochemical-laden selections with purer alternatives, continuing the journey toward healthful living.

## Seemingly Harmless Products

In our previous look into the unseen threats lurking within our food, parasites, and mycotoxins emerged as significant adversaries to our well-being. But as we shift our gaze, it's crucial to recognize that these dangers extend beyond our plates and into the personal products we trust daily, like toothpaste, hair dye, and shampoo. These items, much like our food, carry a veneer of safety and necessity, yet conceal chemicals that pose genuine risks to our health. The glaring gap between cultivated perceptions of safety and the reality of potential harm invites scrutiny, compelling us to unveil these hidden threats.

Every morning, millions of us squeeze a familiar tube of toothpaste, trusting it to nurture dental health. However, many conventional and even some 'natural' toothpaste brands have come under fire for including harmful chemicals. The Cornucopia Institute highlights how products marketed as "natural" often harbor ingredients like carrageenan, which can lead to inflammation, diabetes, and even cancer (The Cornucopia Institute, 2016). Toothpaste lubricates the interior of our mouths, one of the body's most absorbent regions, creating significant concern over toxins entering our bloodstream unchecked. With surfactants like sodium lauryl sulfate potentially containing carcinogenic contaminants, what we use to clean our teeth might do more harm than the sugary items it combats (The Cornucopia Institute, 2016).

The cosmetic industry is no different when it comes to creating illusions. Hair dye, for example, offers the promise of transformation and self-expression, yet often at a perilous cost. Many hair products contain chemicals like ammonia, parabens, and peroxide that can irritate the scalp and leach into the body's systems, presenting risks ranging from mild allergic reactions to potential links with more severe health issues like cancer (Alnuqaydan, 2024). As people pursue beauty standards influenced by social media, the repeated use of these products can lead to an accumulation of toxic substances that affect not just personal health but also the environment. These consequences highlight a discomforting paradox—our desire to appear vibrant leads us to repeated engagements with substances that erode our well-being.

Shampoos, too, serve as a consistent point of contact for introducing harmful chemicals. The saccharine scent and silky promise mask the sinister toxic agents that compose them. Shampoos often contain ingredients like sodium lauryl sulfate, known to cause scalp irritation, and parabens, which mimic body hormones disrupting endocrine systems (Alnuqaydan, 2024; The Cornucopia Institute, 2016). The fact that these ingredients are staples in household brands should serve as a cautionary tale, not just for consumers, but for regulatory bodies as well. Despite the seeming oversight of the FDA, where certain harmful chemicals such as chloroform and mercury compounds are banned, loopholes remain, allowing manufacturers to utilize other hazardous ingredients (Alnuqaydan, 2024).

Consumer trust rests upon the belief that regulations ensure safety, yet, ironically, these very standards often fall short. Regulatory weaknesses and loopholes allow questionable ingredients in personal care products. While legislative efforts, like The Personal Care Products Safety Act, aim to impose stricter evaluations of chemicals used in these products, it's clear that achieving a toxin-free marketplace remains an uphill battle (The Cornucopia Institute, 2016). Until substantial changes take effect, consumers shoulder the burden of navigating these opaque waters.

The broader implications of our cumulative exposure to such everyday toxins resonate beyond mere individual health concerns. As these harmful substances wash down the drain, they mingle with industrial effluents, contributing to environmental pollution. Research underscores the presence of heavy metals like arsenic and lead from these products in wastewater, posing further ecological and public health risks (Alnuqaydan, 2024). The integration of such ingredients into daily routines not only affects users but ultimately traces a detrimental path into the broader ecosystem.

The effects observed are not limited to superficial irritations. We confront a spectrum of potential health complications, from hormone disruption to cancer—a dire consequence of prolonged toxic exposure. Ingredients like formaldehyde, prevalent in nail polishes and hair straighteners, and identified as a carcinogen, call attention to the forgotten reality that what is applied externally seeps into our internal systems, disrupting natural processes and fostering disease (Alnuqaydan, 2024).

As awareness grows, there is a rising clamoring for accountability and reform. Consider the advocacy led by organizations spotlighting toxic toothpastes. Their efforts in creating online resources and scorecards assist conscientious consumers in seeing past marketing guises to make informed choices (The Cornucopia Institute, 2016). This signifies a crucial step toward empowering individuals and holding brands accountable.

The unsettling reality is, our drive for aesthetic and hygienic perfection invites compromised health—a stark contradiction underscoring modern beauty culture's risks. Scrutinizing these everyday products risks highlighting the dire need for transparency and rigorous oversight to ensure safety.

As we peel back layers of concealment from the products we rely upon, our journey now turns to toxic dentistry practices. Just as we assess risks from carcinogens in personal care items, it's imperative to scrutinize dental treatments like root canals and mercury amalgams. This next step will explore the perils of these routine dental practices, continuing our pursuit of truth and transparency in health and wellness.

# Toxic Dentistry

In our daily routines, we often overlook the seemingly harmless practices that disguise potential dangers to our health. We've already explored how common products like toothpaste and shampoo can contain carcinogenic substances. This chapter transitions to dental practices, unveiling the health threats posed by procedures like root canals, mercury amalgams, and dental cavitations.

Root canals might sound routine, yet they harbor hidden risks. These procedures often leave behind infected tissues, which can lead to bacterial infections not just in the mouth but potentially affecting other bodily systems. Dr. Hal Huggins dedicated his career to understanding how root canals could influence overall health, revealing alarming traces of anaerobic bacteria in many tested teeth, thereby establishing a connection between oral infections and systemic health issues (Woods, 2015). His findings suggest that these bacteria, left unchecked within dead teeth, have the potential to migrate throughout the body, causing unforeseen diseases. The implications of Dr. Clark's' research highlight a substantial gap in our understanding of the full effects of root canal procedures.

Similarly, the conversation around mercury amalgams has intensified over the years. Despite longstanding claims of their safety, mounting evidence points to potential dangers associated with mercury exposure. The amalgam fillings used in dental practices contain about 50% mercury, and concerns have risen over mercury's neurotoxic effects. In fact, studies suggest that the mercury in amalgams may leak, posing a risk to the patient's health including breast cancer patients. Dr. Clark's' controversial stance on this issue, supported by blood chemistry analyses, unveiled that removal of mercury fillings often led to dramatic improvements in patient health (Woods, 2015). This directly challenges historical notions held by major dental organizations that have long since dismissed such claims. The inconsistency between believing amalgam is harmless in the mouth, yet toxic when improperly disposed of, points to an irony that draws skepticism and demands further investigation.

Dental cavitations, often overlooked, present another serious concern. These jawbone infections, which linger silently as voids in areas where teeth have been extracted, can contribute to broader health issues. Unseen and untreated, these infections can spread, impacting other areas of health unknowingly. These cavitations may explain unresolved health problems for patients despite ongoing conventional medical care. Dr. Clark's initiative to educate both medical and dental practitioners underscores the importance of recognizing how potential infections can influence overall wellness (Woods, 2015). It emphasizes the need for vigilant monitoring and consideration of alternative diagnostic tools, serving as a reminder of the complexities hidden within routine dental work.

There is no one-size-fits-all solution to addressing these dental concerns. As the industry gradually shifts from mercury amalgams to alternative materials due to instruments like the Minamata Convention, it's clear that patient-specific approaches are critical. Notably, alternatives such as resin-based composites and glass ionomer cements bring their own risks and require informed patient consent and individualized assessments (Schmalz et al., 2023). A broad phase-down of mercury use is already in motion, with more stringent rules progressively being implemented when it comes to its application, particularly in vulnerable groups including children and pregnant women (Schmalz et al., 2023).

The connection between dental practices and systemic health underscores the need for a patient-centered approach. For patients with special needs or higher caries risk, tailored care strategies that include thorough prevention programs are essential. The acknowledgment of personal health risk factors could aid in determining the most effective materials and procedures to minimize adverse outcomes (Schmalz et al., 2023).

Concrete examples of these hidden connections lie in the stories of those like Dr. Weston Price, whose research from decades ago already began hinting at the intricate links between dental health and broader bodily ailments (Woods, 2015). Likewise, personal anecdotes from patients who experienced significant health improvements post-removal of mercury fillings provide a compelling narrative that calls for more awareness and precaution in dental care.

Furthermore, the advancements in understanding dental materials highlight an underlying quest for safer, more biocompatible options in dentistry. Clark's biocompatibility test initiative is one such example, aiming to tailor dental materials to individual patient profiles based on blood chemistry results. This not only enhances the overall safety and effectiveness of dental treatments but also marks a pivotal shift towards integrating personalized medicine into dental practice (Woods, 2015).

As we move beyond the checkpoints of traditional dental assessments, the role of novel diagnostic tools like the Syncrometer becomes relevant. It can detect hidden problems that standard medical tests often miss, offering a broader perspective on ensuring holistic health. This bridge towards advanced diagnostics emphasizes the ongoing importance of comprehensive safety in medical practices, not just for the immediate dental health but also for long-term systemic well-being.

In a rapidly evolving medical landscape, the pursuit of truth and health safety remains paramount. Through continued education and adoption of personalized, innovative approaches, we can better safeguard against the covert risks embedded in our healthcare practices. As we further delve into emerging technologies and methodologies, we reaffirm our commitment to uncovering hidden dangers and guiding toward safer, well-rounded health frameworks.

# Syncrometer Discoveries

Medical scrutiny on dental practices often overlooks potential threats hidden in treatments considered routine. Take root canals, mercury amalgams, and dental cavitations, for instance. Many see these as tried-and-true methods, but concerns have arisen over the less obvious risks they present to health. Root canals, although meant to salvage teeth, can leave behind bacteria that might compromise systemic health. Mercury amalgams, while durable, release mercury vapors over time, potentially affecting brain and kidney functions (Team, 2008). Dental cavitations, voids in jawbones that sometimes accompany wisdom tooth extractions, can harbor pathogens that standard X-rays might miss. This cloud of undetectable issues sets the stage for alternative diagnostic approaches like the Syncrometer.

Developed outside the usual medical paradigm, the Syncrometer claims to identify threats conventional tools might leave unrecognized. While mainstream practitioners base diagnostics on visible symptoms and lab tests, the Syncrometer purportedly detects the presence of pathogens, toxins, and pollutants through an unorthodox electrical resonance technique (Swiss company charged by FTC with making unsubstantiated health claims, 2003). Critics often point out the lack of empirical data supporting the device's efficacy; however, its proponents argue that it fills gaps left by traditional medical practices. This tool, stationed in the margins of science, underscores the notion that hidden threats exist even in a world heavily charted by medical progress.

Consider environmental toxins in household items, a prime example of hidden dangers the Syncrometer might bring to light. Everyday products like cleaning agents and air fresheners often contain volatile organic compounds (VOCs) that contribute to chronic respiratory and neurological illnesses. Most health practitioners focus on allergens while treating patients with respiratory issues, potentially ignoring VOCs, which are unseen and seldom discussed. Even toys and electronics emit flame retardants that can act as endocrine disruptors, subtly influencing hormonal balance over time. The Syncrometer, according to its supporters, pinpoints these clandestine aggressors in ways traditional diagnostics might not, suggesting a need for broader awareness of environmental health (Team, 2008).

Let's explore the potential impact of dietary supplements, another domain fraught with obscured health risks. Supplements, often marketed with grand claims of providing essential nutrients, sometimes contain unregulated substances. For instance, certain weight loss supplements might include stimulants not disclosed on labels, contributing to hypertension or kidney issues. Although regulatory bodies like the FDA monitor these products, gaps in oversight mean some risks fly under the radar. Not bound by such restrictions, the Syncrometer supposedly uncovers harmful ingredients by assessing their energetic frequencies, presenting a critique of current regulatory efficacy (Swiss company charged by FTC with making unsubstantiated health claims, 2003).

Beyond supplements, consider the pollutants from nearby industries, a hazard often invisible to nearby residents. Factories can release heavy metals and airborne chemicals that settle into local environments, infiltrating water supplies and local food chains. Over time, these pollutants may contribute to chronic conditions like cancer or neurodegenerative diseases. Traditional diagnostics, focusing primarily on symptomatic relief, might overlook this community-level exposure. Proponents of the Syncrometer argue its sensitivity to these contaminants could complement existing environmental health assessments, broadening our understanding of population health impacts.

Yet, we should approach such claims with critical thinking. The medical field requires rigorous scrutiny to protect patient safety, but existing frameworks might lack the capacity to explore every environmental variable influencing health. For example, noise pollution, an often underappreciated factor, can increase stress and cardiovascular risks. It's a threat that's difficult to quantify with existing diagnostic criteria but affects wellbeing nonetheless. The Syncrometer's purported ability to detect stress frequencies from noise offers a novel perspective, albeit one lacking empirical substantiation (Team, 2008).

However, addressing hidden health threats isn't just about pointing out unseen dangers. It involves broadening public and professional awareness, enhancing diagnostic capabilities to recognize these threats. The Syncrometer, while controversial, sparks discussion on areas where medical science might lag. Continuing debates encourage innovation and deeper inquiry into environmental and microbial factors affecting health, fostering a more holistic approach to wellness (Swiss company charged by FTC with making unsubstantiated health claims, 2003).

Moreover, personal choices amplify these hidden risks. Consider dietary habits, where processed foods high in sugar and additives contribute to obesity and diabetes. Routine blood tests capture the biochemical aftermath of poor diet choices, yet they don't necessarily trace back to the micro-level dietary contributors like preservatives and artificial sweeteners. Detecting these acute dietary threats requires nuanced tools beyond the traditional scope. The Syncrometer's advocates propose it can discern these overlooked culprits, challenging established nutritional pathology norms.

We should also acknowledge the psychosocial contexts influencing health beyond biochemical markers. Chronic stress, often overlooked, plays a significant role in the progression of diseases. Stressors from modern life mount cumulatively, and traditional diagnostics might not capture their pervasive influence. The Syncrometer's proponents suggest it identifies these energetic stress imbalances, even if current medical technologies concentrate more on physiological than psychological factors (Team, 2008).

Ultimately, the Syncrometer's narratives of discovery prompt reevaluation of what it means to truly understand health risks. While skepticism lingers around its claims, the conversation it fosters encourages deeper exploration of how modern life quietly shapes health outcomes. It's a reminder of the constant evolution of medical science, where inquiry and innovation explore beyond visible horizons. By engaging with these contentious ideas, we strive for a healthcare future that's more aware, more responsive, and more inclusive of the nuanced ways our environments and lifestyles influence health.

# Concluding Thoughts

Having explored the hidden dangers in our everyday food supply, it's clear that understanding these risks is crucial for protecting our health. The presence of parasites, mycotoxins, azo dyes, and heavy metals in what we eat underscores a larger issue of pervasive contaminants threatening our well-being every day. As consumers, we now possess the knowledge to challenge conventional systems and demand transparency, pushing for cleaner, safer alternatives in our diets. This awareness beckons us to embrace mindful consumerism, advocating for transparent labeling and sustainable practices that can lead to healthier choices. By leveraging this insight, we can collectively drive change toward reducing exposure to these hidden threats, promoting wellness not just in individual lives but across communities. Through informed decisions and proactive advocacy, we have the power to mitigate these dangers and contribute to a future where our food and personal products support rather than hinder our health.

# Conclusion

In a world increasingly drawn to alternative healing, Dr. Clark's story offers a poignant reflection on the challenges faced by those who dare to deviate from conventional medical paths. Her protocol, grounded in natural remedies and holistic techniques, has become a beacon for many seeking empowerment over their health journeys. Yet, despite the apparent success stories, her work faced relentless skepticism and resistance from the mainstream medical community—a powerful reminder of the systemic barriers that often hinder innovative treatments.

For those who already embrace alternative medicines—whether through herbal therapies, detox regimens, or energy healing—the appeal of Dr. Clark's methods is clear. These individuals often find solace in natural cures, seeking alternatives that resonate with their bodies' innate healing capabilities. The promise of self-healing and medical freedom is especially alluring to communities conversant with platforms like Facebook groups and YouTube channels dedicated to holistic wellness. Dr. Clark's protocol represents a lifeline for these seekers, offering a route to health that honors both traditional wisdom and modern needs without relying exclusively on pharmaceutical interventions.

However, the path to integrating such alternatives into recognized healthcare models is fraught with obstacles. Regulatory frameworks and entrenched ideologies within the healthcare system often create an environment that marginalizes non-traditional methods. Critics are quick to dismiss them as fringe science, overlooking mounting evidence and patient testimonials that speak to their efficacy. This skepticism is exacerbated by vested interests keen to maintain the status quo, safeguarding established revenue streams over revolutionary approaches.

For medical freedom advocates, this narrative echoes prevalent fears surrounding autonomy and systemic control. Skeptical of mainstream medicine and wary of perceived overreach by entities like the FDA and CDC, these individuals value bodily autonomy above all else. Platforms like X (Twitter) and podcasts with figures such as RFK Jr. serve as crucial arenas where they voice concerns about censorship and advocate for unrestricted access to diverse treatment options.

Among chronic illness sufferers and cancer survivors, Dr. Clark's methods offer a glimmer of hope. Many have journeyed through the labyrinth of conventional medicine only to find themselves at a dead-end, still plagued by unresolved conditions. For them, the potential of alternative treatments signifies not just relief but a chance at redemption—a testament to the human spirit's resilience when confronted with seemingly insurmountable health challenges. They turn to online forums and social media threads to share experiences, fostering communities of support and shared knowledge that transcend geographical boundaries.

Similarly, those who dwell on the fringes of societal norms—the truth seekers deeply skeptical of governmental transparency—find resonance in Clark's tale. This group thrives on uncovering hidden truths, questioning the narratives put forth by mainstream institutions, and exploring theories about global suppression of life-saving innovations. In their quest for understanding, they challenge the narratives imposed by society, advocating for recognition of overlooked remedies and questioning why certain protocols face suppression.

In unifying these distinct audiences, Dr. Clark's story highlights a common pursuit: the quest for truth in healing. Her protocol transcends mere treatment, becoming a rallying cry for patient empowerment. By granting individuals access to genuine information, it enables them to navigate beyond the constraints of conventional practices, fostering a culture of inquiry and liberation.

Amidst this exploration lies a broader conversation on the systemic inadequacies of our current medical framework. The inertia ingrained within these structures often poses the most formidable challenge to transformative change, impeding the adoption of potentially groundbreaking protocols like Clark's. Financial constraints, regulatory hurdles, and ideological biases converge to form a resistant barrier to innovation. To bridge these divides, a collective shift is required—one that values transparency, inclusivity, and patient-centered healthcare.

Dr. Clark's narrative illustrates the power of embracing diverse healing paths, challenging us to reconsider what constitutes valid medical practice. Empowered patients must actively participate in reshaping this landscape, demanding systems that honor their right to explore alternative treatments without bias or restriction. Whether through advocacy or personal journeys toward wellness, the call for transformation reverberates across society, urging a reevaluation of how we perceive health and care.

As we stand at the crossroads of possibility, it becomes imperative to dismantle the barriers that stifle innovation. A new era of healthcare beckons—one that integrates holistic methodologies with technological advancements, promoting an ecosystem where traditional and unconventional treatments coexist harmoniously. It demands open dialogue among practitioners, policymakers, and patients alike, paving the way for a future where all voices are heard and valued.

Ultimately, Dr. Clark's protocol symbolizes the potential for change within a rigid healthcare system. It invites us to embrace inquiry and curiosity, championing the rights of individuals to chart their healing paths. By fostering environments of openness and understanding, we can transform healthcare into an inclusive space where diversity of thought leads to comprehensive wellness solutions. Through collaboration and a shared commitment to progress, a more responsive and empowering system awaits, ready to accommodate the varied needs of its constituents.

# Appendices

Have you ever wondered how a single idea could alter the landscape of health and medicine? Dr. Clark's contributions to holistic health have sparked not just curiosity but also debate and intrigue. For many, her methods present an alternative path to wellness, shunning the mainstream in favor of natural self-healing techniques. Yet, with groundbreaking ideas often comes controversy, mixed receptions, and the challenge of finding acceptance within established structures. Consider the stories that surface—testimonials from those who have found relief through her protocols juxtaposed against legal battles questioning their validity.

This chapter delves into the intricate mosaic of Dr. Clark's journey, encapsulating the personal and societal impacts of her work. From the heartfelt testimonials sharing life-changing experiences to the scrutiny faced in courtrooms, these narratives provide a comprehensive view of the influence and challenges encountered by pioneers in alternative health. As we explore these dimensions, you'll gain insight into how individual testimonies intertwine with broader societal dynamics and legal frameworks, setting the stage for further discussions on the integration of Dr. Clark's methods into diverse medical practices worldwide.

# Testimonials and Legal Battles

From the previous discussion of Dr. Clark's holistic health protocols, we move into a realm where testimonials and legal challenges intersect to provide richer insights. This section aims to bridge personal experiences and societal reactions, bringing to light the influence of Dr. Clark's work on individuals and institutions.

Real-life testimonials bear witness to the efficacy and reach of Dr. Clark's methods. Take Anna's story, for instance. Struggling with chronic fatigue, Anna embarked on Dr. Clark's Parasite Protocol. Within weeks, she reported feeling energized and revitalized. Her testimony underscores the potential these alternative methods hold for individuals seeking solutions traditional medicine seemed unable to provide.

In parallel, consider the journey of Michael, who battled recurring kidney stones. Through consistent application of the Kidney Cleanse, he found relief and a new lease on life. Michael's account adds to a collective narrative that suggests a tangible impact on personal health struggles. These stories, though varied, highlight a shared theme of empowerment and transformation enabled by Dr. Clark's protocols. Testimonials such as these form a tapestry of narratives that reinforce the practical outcomes of the methods previously discussed.

However, the journey of these alternative practices also winds its way through the corridors of legal scrutiny. At the heart of these legal battles lies the tension between innovation and regulation. Dr. Clark faced numerous legal challenges, reflecting broader societal attitudes toward non-conventional practices. These incidents did more than scrutinize the validity of her methods; they spotlighted shifting power dynamics and a growing curiosity about alternative health solutions.

Consider the 1993 ruling in the case of State v. Michaels. Although not directly related to Dr. Clark, this case exemplifies how legal systems can challenge evidence derived from flawed methodologies (Howe & Knott, 2015). The reversal of convictions based on unreliable child testimonies due to coercive interview techniques reminded advocates of all forms that methodologies matter, whether in law or health. This precedent underscored the need for reputation and rigor in unconventional areas, including alternative health practices.

Dr. Clark's legal battles, though centered on her specific protocols, mirrored this broader societal dynamic. As her methods gained traction, so too did skepticism and legal pushback. These proceedings often reflected a clash between established medical institutions and emerging alternative paradigms. In several instances, the legal outcomes forced a reevaluation of what constituted evidence and expertise within the health domain.

The narrative arc of these legal confrontations reveals much about the era's perception of alternative medicine. During the 1990s, a noticeable pivot occurred. The fraying trust in established medical systems, chronicled extensively by scholars like Tracey E. George, began pushing more individuals toward empirical, yet non-traditional health research (Salehijam, 2018). Dr. Clark's legal journeys unfolded within this context of shifting perceptions and rising challenges, providing a backdrop for a broader conversation about autonomy, choice, and evidence.

Piecing together these legal timelines helps situate Dr. Clark's contributions within a larger framework. The catalytic moments in these legal battles were not solely about legality but spoke to a deeper judiciary acknowledgment of alternative approaches gaining traction among the populace. Each courtroom decision did not just affect Dr. Clark but echoed throughout the larger alternative health community, encouraging more practitioners to pursue avenues that were once considered unconventional.

From the initial controversies to wider acknowledgment of her methods' validity, the timeline of legal battles illustrates the resilience required to introduce novel ideas into the mainstream. These events were less about contesting her methods and more about testing an established system's flexibility to entertain new methodologies. They subsequently prompted a reevaluation and gradual acceptance of complementary and alternative medicine by established health systems.

As we gather these testimonials and narratives of legal scrutiny, they not only enrich our understanding but also set the stage for what follows. The personal stories and courtroom dramas meld into a narrative that highlights the persistence and potential pitfalls of pioneering work. They pave the way for acknowledgment and adaptation by healthcare professionals and medical institutions.

Transitioning forward, this context becomes crucial for understanding the adoption of Dr. Clark's methods by various practitioners and clinics. This evolution from personal narratives to professional validation underscores a growing acknowledgment of her approach, which eventually found its way into the broader spheres of clinical application. Through this lens, we see how patient experiences and legal considerations weave into the professional fabric, marking a transition from personal advocacy to institutional practice.

Looking ahead, the forthcoming section will introduce readers to a list of doctors and clinics that have embraced Dr. Clark's methodologies. This transition from testimonials and legal histories to professional adoption highlights the convergence of personal conviction with formalized medical practice.

As this discussion flows seamlessly into more professional aspects, the narrative arc—from personal, to legal, to professional—encapsulates a journey of acceptance, underscoring the growing validation and continued influence of Dr. Clark's work in various healthcare settings. This transition prepares readers for an exploration of how her methods continue to thrive in professional spheres, offering further illumination on an ever-evolving landscape of health.

# Doctors and Clinics

Previously, we explored the personal accounts and legal challenges that framed Dr. Clark's journey. Now, these narratives take on a broader dimension as we delve into the substantial influence her methods have etched in the fabric of alternative medicine, specifically through the adoption by doctors and clinics worldwide. These endorsements serve as testaments to the efficacy and respect her approaches have garnered, often transcending geographical and cultural boundaries to find a home in diverse medical practices.

Many practitioners initially drawn to Dr. Clark's methods were inspired by their holistic approach. Holistic medicine views the body as an interconnected whole rather than a sum of isolated parts, a philosophy that aligns well with Dr. Clark's focus on treating the underlying causes rather than just symptoms, as articulated in Cleveland Clinic's overview of what defines a holistic perspective (What Is a Holistic Doctor & Where Can I Find One?, n.d.). This principle resonates with numerous healthcare providers seeking to offer their patients more comprehensive care.

In Ohio, Dr. Wilson, a well-known osteopathic doctor, adopts Clark's methodologies to provide integrative health solutions. A prominent figure in holistic healthcare, Dr. Wilson emphasizes preventative care and patient empowerment. He treats a wide array of conditions by integrating Clark's techniques, especially her unique views on toxin elimination and nutrition. His patients often report significant improvements in chronic conditions such as autoimmune diseases and allergies, showcasing a tangible testament to the effectiveness of Dr. Clark's methods.

Dr. Emily Chen, practicing in an integrative center in Toronto, is another practitioner who has embraced these approaches. Dr. Chen's clinic sees a diverse clientele, from individuals recovering from complex surgeries to those managing mental health conditions. Her adoption of Dr. Clark's protocols, particularly those addressing environmental toxins, reflects her commitment to exploring all avenues for comprehensive patient care. Her success stories include a young patient overcoming persistent fatigue and an elderly woman achieving improved mobility after adopting Dr. Clark's guidance on detoxification and cellular health.

Venturing into Europe, Dr. Karlsson in Stockholm is renowned for blending traditional chiropractic techniques with Dr. Clark's holistic principles. Dr. Karlsson focuses on the interconnection between musculoskeletal health and other bodily systems. His innovative approach has attracted many patients with chronic pain issues, who praise his methods for their holistic benefits that go beyond mere symptom alleviation.

These practitioners reflect a growing interest in models of care that value the balance of body and mind—a core tenet of holistic medicine as seen with many holistic doctors globally (What Is a Holistic Doctor & Where Can I Find One?, n.d.). Clinics from various parts of the world actively incorporate Dr. Clark's methods into their practice despite geographical differences.

Incorporating these techniques often involves a transition that requires re-education and a shift in mindset for practitioners. Many cite increased patient satisfaction and improved health outcomes as key motivators. This transition to holistic treatment has been complemented by the rise of telemedicine, which has offered tools for remote consultations and follow-ups, further spreading the reach of these protocols (Use of Telemedicine among Office-Based Physicians, 2021 | HealthIT.gov, n.d.).

The integration of telemedicine has significantly impacted the availability of Dr. Clark's methods across underserved or rural areas. A noteworthy example is in remote parts of Australia, where practitioners utilize telemedicine to consult with patients otherwise unable to access specialized holistic healthcare. Telemedicine not only broadens access but also allows for continuous patient engagement, which is pivotal in maintaining holistic healthcare outcomes (Use of Telemedicine among Office-Based Physicians, 2021 | HealthIT.gov, n.d.).

These stories underscore a network of adoption that strengthens the legitimacy of Dr. Clark's work. The openness to alternative methods speaks volumes about the growing acceptance of diverse medical practices that look beyond conventional treatments. It highlights a shift toward integrative health solutions that consider medical, emotional, and lifestyle factors, embodying a holistic approach that can lead to more profound and lasting health benefits.

As we move toward the concluding sections of this chapter, the upcoming content will anchor these narratives in robust foundational references, detailing the research and citations that underpin Dr. Clark's methodologies. This serves to further validate the approaches taken by compassionate and exploratory practitioners worldwide. By weaving together personal experiences, legal narratives, and professional adoption, readers gain a rich tapestry of how Dr. Clark's legacy is carried forward in modern healthcare, powering a movement that champions patient-centered, holistic healing practices revered across the globe.

# Research Acknowledgments

In looking at the application of Dr. Hulda Clark's methods by various healthcare professionals and clinics, we see an intersection of theory and practice that highlights both the opportunities and challenges of alternative health approaches. These practitioners provide a strong foundation of practical evidence supporting the principles Clark laid out, bridging the gap between her theories and real-world applications. The meticulous documentation these professionals maintained plays a critical role in reinforcing Dr. Clark's protocols through credible sources and citations. This link between practice and scholarly evidence not only validates the effectiveness but also advances the credibility of alternative medicine within mainstream dialogues (Lyons, n.d.).

In the contested realm of alternative health, where Dr. Clark's methodologies reside, citing reliable data stands as an essential pillar for ensuring trust and authenticity. The practice of integrating peer-reviewed journal articles, clinical trials, and documented case studies provides substantial weight to the claims. Resources like these demonstrate that her methods have not just been acknowledged but also strategically deployed to achieve desired health outcomes among diverse populations (Kingsley, 2022). For instance, looking toward studies where Dr. Clark's protocols were a focal point can illuminate how they challenge conventional medical narratives by providing alternate avenues for treatment. Such references are pivotal as they lend authority and validation to often-overlooked practices.

Consider the situation where health seekers, skeptical of mainstream practices, turn to forums and publications discussing Dr. Clark's methods. The specificity and reliability of sources used in these publications greatly influence their reception. When these discussions include in-text citations of peer-reviewed articles or reports from reputable institutions, they reflect thorough research and professionalism that assist individuals in making informed decisions (Lyons, n.d.). Consequently, independent sources not only bolster the persuasive power of the text but also illustrate the diversity of thought and evidence within the landscape of health and wellness.

Moreover, using distinct examples of these resources consolidates support for Dr. Clark's protocols. When peer-reviewed studies are cited alongside anecdotal evidence and case reports, they combine to offer a more holistic picture of efficacy. The convergence of narrative testimony with scientific inquiry speaks to a deeper truth: alternative health, while often dismissed, is grounded in both experiential and empirical realities. The interplay between these elements creates a comprehensive narrative not easy to dismiss, even by staunch critics of alternative methodologies (Kingsley, 2022).

Credible citations and the careful documentation of sources exhibit the rigor and depth of research that underpin Dr. Clark's methods. By clearly presenting the origins of these ideas and the outcomes observed in practice, practitioners make a case for a broader understanding and acceptance of alternative measures. The meticulous nature of citation also serves to educate and inform, allowing audiences to further explore validated studies and outcomes that support or challenge Dr. Clark's claims. This openness and transparency, embodied in detailed sourcing, signify respect for both the knowledge that precedes us and the discoveries we seek to make our own.

Furthermore, emphasizing peer-reviewed and independent sources underscores the importance of impartiality and consensus across disciplines when evaluating the merit of alternative protocols. Such inclusion of a broad spectrum of perspectives nudges the conversation from a polarized standpoint toward a more nuanced analysis that resonates with inquisitive and critical thinkers. By rigorously citing and documenting these sources, the argument for alternative health maintains its respectability, positioning it within a professional and ethical framework respected by students and scholars alike (Lyons, n.d.).

In sum, the act of thorough citation accomplishes more than adherence to scholarly etiquette; it signals a commitment to truth and fairness within the discourse. As practitioners and scholars lend credence to Dr. Clark's methods through careful citation, they don't just reinforce existing beliefs but invite new dialogues and discoveries that may redefine the parameters of health and wellness. The impact is profound: promoting trust, facilitating education, and encouraging a collaborative effort between traditional and alternative health paradigms.

In navigating this contested space, the employment of credible sources and citations becomes not merely a scholarly exercise but a foundational strategy in constructing a narrative that strives for acceptance across ideological divides.

By valuing Dr. Clark's insights and those of her contemporaries with rigorous citation, practitioners and readers alike create a robust repository of knowledge that supports alternative methods while enriching the broader field of healthcare discourse.

## Concluding Thoughts

Dr. Clark's contributions to holistic health, marked by both personal testimonials and legal challenges, reveal a complex narrative of innovation and resilience. Her protocols have sparked significant interest, with stories from individuals like Anna and Michael showcasing their transformative potential. However, the path has not been entirely smooth, as societal skepticism and legal scrutiny highlight the tension between emerging alternative practices and established medical norms. These narratives underline a pivotal era where alternative medicine gained traction amidst growing dissatisfaction with conventional treatments. Looking forward, the integration of her methods by practitioners worldwide hints at an evolving landscape where alternative solutions are increasingly embraced in healthcare. As we understand the depth and impact of Dr. Clark's work, we find ourselves poised to explore its growing acceptance among doctors and clinics, forming a bridge from individual experiences to broader institutional practice. This journey encourages us to consider how these approaches might redefine health paradigms and inspire pathways for future explorations into patient-centered healing.

# Timeline of Dr. Hulda Clark's Life & Activities

**1928 – Birth**

- Dr. Hulda Regehr Clark is born on October 18, 1928, in Saskatchewan, Canada.

**1950s–1960s – Academic Training**

- Earns a **Bachelor of Arts** and **Master's degree** in biology.
- Receives a **Ph.D. in physiology** from the University of Minnesota.
- Conducts postdoctoral work in cell physiology.

**1970s–1980s – Alternative Research Begins**

- Begins to question mainstream medicine and shifts toward independent research.
- Studies **nutrition, herbal remedies, and electronic frequencies.**
- Develops what later becomes the **"Clark Zapper"**, a low-voltage frequency device she claims kills parasites and bacteria.

**1993 – Publishes First Book**

- Releases *"The Cure for All Cancers"*, which claims that cancer is caused by parasites and toxins and that it can be cured through detoxification and the zapper.
- Book generates controversy and gains underground popularity in natural health circles.

**1995–2000 – Mainstream Pushback**

- Publishes additional books:
    - *The Cure for HIV and AIDS*
    - *The Cure for All Diseases*

    - *The Cure for Advanced Cancers*
- Draws criticism from the medical establishment and attention from regulatory agencies.

**1999 – Arrest and Legal Battle**

- **Indiana authorities issue a warrant** for practicing medicine without a license.
- Dr. Clark is **arrested in San Diego, extradited in a police car** across state lines at age 72, and **put on trial.**
- She is **acquitted**—found **not guilty** on all charges.

**2000s – Clinic in Tijuana, Mexico**

- Opens a clinic in **Tijuana**, just across the U.S.–Mexico border, where she treats patients who report having been helped by her detox and parasite-cleansing protocols.
- Continues to lecture, publish, and support holistic therapies.

**2009 – Death**

- **Dr. Hulda Clark dies on September 3, 2009**, reportedly from complications of anemia.
- Critics claim she died of cancer, but this has never been medically confirmed or documented.

**Post-2009 – Legacy and Influence**

- Her books remain widely circulated in alternative health communities.
- Thousands claim that her methods—including **zappers, liver cleanses**, and **parasite protocols**—helped them heal from chronic conditions.
- Advocates compare her to other persecuted alternative healers like **Dr. Sebi, Royal Rife**, and **Max Gerson**.

- A resurgence of interest in her work emerged during COVID-19, as public skepticism of conventional medicine grew.

# Reference List


**Chapter 1 The Woman They Couldn't Ignore**

Chancellor, J., & Lyubomirsky, S. (2013, November). Humble Beginnings: Current Trends, State Perspectives, and Hallmarks of Humility. Social and Personality Psychology Compass. https://doi.org/10.1111/spc3.12069

Does Bio-Resonance really work? | ResearchGate. (2018). ResearchGate. https://www.researchgate.net/post/Does-Bio-Resonance-really-work

Dr. Hulda Clark | The Paramount Zapper. (2024). The Paramount Zapper. https://www.paramountzapper.com/about-3

Durant, J. M., & Allen, J. M. (2024, August 28). My Story... From Humble Beginnings to Professional Success. Taylor & Francis.

Karakos, P., Grigorios, T., Theodoros, K., & Theodoros, L. (2019, April 30). The Effectiveness of Bioresonance Method on Human Health. The Open Epidemiology Journal. https://doi.org/10.2174/1874297120190800001

Lee, E. L., Richards, N., Harrison, J., & Barnes, J. (2022, July). Prevalence of Use of Traditional, Complementary and Alternative Medicine by the General Population: A Systematic Review of National Studies Published from 2010 to 2019. Drug Safety. https://doi.org/10.1007/s40264-022-01189-w

Miller, R. V., & Jr. (2024, February 7). Monsanto Roundup Lawsuit Update. Lawsuit Information Center. https://www.lawsuit-information-center.com/roundup-lawsuit.html

Regulatory, Scientific & Quality Conference | Consumer Healthcare Products Association. (2024). Chpa.org. https://www.chpa.org/events-education/regulatory-scientific-quality-conference

**Chapter 2 Discovering the Root Cause**

Carroll, A. E. (2018, November 5). Peer Review: The Worst Way to Judge Research, Except for All the Others. The New York Times. https://www.nytimes.com/2018/11/05/upshot/peer-review-the-worst-way-to-judge-research-except-for-all-the-others.html

Oskar. (2025, March 18). Nature is always on our side, protecting us in hundreds of ways. Dr. Hulda Clark. https://drhuldaclark.org/nature-is-always-on-our-side-protecting-us-in-hundreds-of-ways/

O'Kelly, E., Cwiklinski, K., De, C., Davies, E., Corrales, J. L., Jewhurst, H., Flaus, A., Lalor, R., Serrat, J., Dalton, J. P., & González-Miguel, J. (2024, August 30). Moonlighting on the Fasciola hepatica tegument: Enolase, a glycolytic enzyme, interacts with the extracellular matrix and fibrinolytic system of the host. PLoS Neglected Tropical Diseases; Public Library of Science. https://doi.org/10.1371/journal.pntd.0012069

Shany-Ur, T., Poorzand, P., Grossman, S. N., Growdon, M. E., Jang, J. Y., Ketelle, R. S., Miller, B. L., & Rankin, K. P. (2012, November). Comprehension of insincere communication in neurodegenerative disease: Lies, sarcasm, and theory of mind. Cortex. https://doi.org/10.1016/j.cortex.2011.08.003

Schantz, P. M., Moore, A. C., Muñoz, J. L., Hartman, B. J., Schaefer, J. A., Aron, A. M., Persaud, D., Sarti, E., Wilson, M., & Flisser, A. (1992, September 3). Neurocysticercosis in an Orthodox Jewish Community in New York City. New England Journal of Medicine. https://doi.org/10.1056/nejm199209033271004

Saad Motawéa. (2025). The Bizarre Claims of Hulda Clark. Scribd. https://id.scribd.com/document/135718751/The-Bizarre-Claims-of-Hulda-Clark?referrer=utm_campaign%3Dapp_promo%26utm_source%3Dinterstitial%2(

Yu, S. (2010, August 10). Who is Afraid of Hulda Clark? Asymmetric Warfare on Cancer - Prevention & Healing Inc. Prevention & Healing Inc. https://preventionandhealing.com/blog/who-is-afraid-of-hulda-clark-asymmetric-warfare-on-cancer/

Zolfaghari Emameh, R., Purmonen, S., Sukura, A., & Parkkila, S. (2017, November 12). Surveillance and diagnosis of zoonotic foodborne parasites. Food Science & Nutrition. https://doi.org/10.1002/fsn3.530

**Chapter 3 The Zapper, the Cleanses, and the Cure**

NOW Foods Now Foods, (2 Pack) Fresh Green Black Walnut Wormwood Complex, 2 fl oz (60 ml) : Health & Household. (2025). Filipinodoctors.org. https://medicalbooks.filipinodoctors.org/item/B004RRBXYO

Crouse, M. (2015). Inca Medicine: Religion, Culture, and Ethnobotany – Writing Anthology. Central.edu. https://central.edu/writing-anthology/2019/05/29/inca-medicine-religion-culture-and-ethnobotany/

Filipič, B., Rihar, K., Gregorič, D. E., Gradišnik, L., Pereyra, A., Đermić, D., Daničić, Č., & Mazija, H. (2019, January 1). Enhancing Effect of 100.414-kHz Electromagnetic Field Produced by Defender's Pulse Generator on the ChIFN γ-Like Molecule Inducing Capacity of Lens culinaris Agglutinin and 10% PBS Washouts of Different Holocene Minerals. Technology in Cancer Research & Treatment; SAGE Publications. https://doi.org/10.1177/1533033818821093

Metwaly, A. M., Ghoneim, M. M., Eissa, Ibrahim. H., Elsehemy, I. A., Mostafa, A. E., Hegazy, M. M., Afifi, W. M., & Dou, D. (2021, June 19). Traditional Ancient Egyptian Medicine: a Review. Saudi Journal of Biological Sciences. https://doi.org/10.1016/j.sjbs.2021.06.044

Pan, S. C. (n.d.). Research Paper Structure. Psychology.ucsd.edu. https://psychology.ucsd.edu/undergraduate-program/undergraduate-resources/academic-writing-resources/writing-research-papers/research-paper-structure.html

Rife machines and cancer. (n.d.). Www.cancerresearchuk.org. https://www.cancerresearchuk.org/about-cancer/treatment/complementary-alternative-therapies/individual-therapies/rife-machine-and-cancer

Shor, S. M., & Schweig, S. K. (2023, July 1). The Use of Natural Bioactive Nutraceuticals in the Management of Tick-Borne Illnesses. Microorganisms. https://doi.org/10.3390/microorganisms11071759

University of Southern California. (2010). Research Guides: Organizing Your Social Sciences Research Paper: 8. The Discussion. Usc.edu. https://libguides.usc.edu/writingguide/discussion

**Chapter 4 Testimonies From the Healed**

(2016). Iiarjournals.org. https://ar.iiarjournals.org/content/44/9/3725

A Path to Improved Health Care Worker Well-Being: Lessons from the COVID-19 Pandemic - NAM. (2025). NAM. https://nam.edu/perspectives/a-path-to-improved-health-care-worker-well-being-lessons-from-the-covid-19-pandemic/

Ben-Arye, E., Finkelstein, A., Samuels, N., Ben-Yehuda, D., Schiff, E., Reis, S., Lesser, L., Bergel, M., & Shaham, D. (2022, February 10). From skepticism to openness: a qualitative narrative analysis of medical students' attitudes following an integrative medicine course. Supportive Care in Cancer. https://doi.org/10.1007/s00520-022-06888-9

Bay Area Lyme. (2015, November 30). Straight Talk about Biofilms: A New Answer for Treating Lyme Disease? - Bay Area Lyme Foundation. Bay Area Lyme Foundation. https://www.bayarealyme.org/blog/straight-talk-biofilms-new-answer-treating-lyme-disease/

Chai, J.-Y., Jung, B.-K., & Hong, S.-J. (2021, June 1). Albendazole and Mebendazole as Anti-Parasitic and Anti-Cancer Agents: an Update. The Korean Journal of Parasitology. https://doi.org/10.3347/kjp.2021.59.3.189

FTC v. Dr. Clark Research Association - Complaint. (2025). Ftc.gov. https://www.ftc.gov/sites/default/files/documents/cases/2003/01/030127comp0223051.shtm

Hulda Clark's "zapper" device is based on pseudoscience; doesn't kill parasites or cure diseases - Science Feedback. (2024, January 12). Science Feedback. https://science.feedback.org/review/hulda-clarks-zapper-device-is-based-on-pseudoscience-doesnt-kill-parasites-or-cure-diseases/

Press, D. (2025). Search result for "Evidence-." Dovepress.com. https://www.dovepress.com/search_results.php?search_word=Evidence-

**Chapter 5 Standing Trial for Curing People**

Criminal Convictions and Medical Licensure. (2011, October 1). AMA Journal of Ethics. https://doi.org/10.1001/virtualmentor.2011.13.10.pfor1-1110

Glass, L. T., Schlachta, C. M., Hawel, J. D., Elnahas, A. I., & Alkhamesi, N. A. (2022, December). Cross-border healthcare: A review and applicability to North America during COVID-19. Health Policy OPEN. https://doi.org/10.1016/j.hpopen.2021.100064

How Should Clinicians Express Solidarity With Asylum Seekers at the US-Mexico Border? (2022, April 1). AMA Journal of Ethics. https://doi.org/10.1001/amajethics.2022.275

IMLA Legal Advocacy Program. (2025, January 7). IMLA. https://imla.org/legal-advocacy/

Medical News. (1903, March 7). https://doi.org/10.1001/jama.1903.02490100036007

Territoriality in American Criminal Law - Michigan Law Review. (2023, June 27). Michigan Law Review. https://michiganlawreview.org/journal/territoriality-in-american-criminal-law/

The 21st Century Cures Act and Information Blocking. (2016). MagMutual. https://www.magmutual.com/healthcare-insights/article/21st-century-cures-act-and-information-blocking

Wong, H. (2020, May 15). The case for compulsory licensing during COVID-19. Journal of Global Health. https://doi.org/10.7189/jogh.10.010358

**Chapter 6 The global Movement She Sparked**

Clubs.dir.bg. http://clubs.dir.bg/showflat.php?Board=rak&Number=1951704680&page=&view=&a

Dr. Clark Research Association, Dr. Clark Behandlungzentrum GMbH, d/b/a Dr. Clark Zentrum, and David P. Amrein. (2004, November 30). Federal Trade Commission. https://www.ftc.gov/legal-library/browse/cases-proceedings/022-3165-dr-clark-research-association-dr-clark-behandlungzentrum-gmbh-dba-dr-clark-zentrum-david-p-amrein

Dr. Clark Store | The Leader In Pure Vitamins and Supplements. (2025, April 29). Dr. Clark Store. https://www.curezone.org/a.asp?i=662

Full text of "CLEANSING THERAPY - CURE YOURSELF." (2016). Archive.org. https://archive.org/stream/cy-book/cy-book_djvu.txt

FTC v. Dr. Clark Research Association - Complaint. (2025). Ftc.gov. https://www.ftc.gov/sites/default/files/documents/cases/2003/01/030127comp0223051.shtm

The Cardinals of the Holy Roman Church - Additions 2015. (2015). Fiu.edu. http://cardinals.fiu.edu/additions-15.htm

Yumpu.com. (2015). Physiology/Pharmacology - ARVO. Yumpu.com. https://www.yumpu.com/en/document/view/41472593/physiology-pharmacology-arvo

**Chapter 7 If She Was Wrong, Why Were People Getting Healed?**

Admin. (2021, March 23). Sick and tired: How the medical field neglects women's health. The Tribune. https://www.thetribune.ca/sci-tech/sick-and-tired-how-the-medical-field-neglects-womens-health-03232021/

Boden, L. I., & Ozonoff, D. (2008, January). Litigation-Generated Science: Why Should We Care? Environmental Health Perspectives. https://doi.org/10.1289/ehp.9987

Iragorri, N., de Oliveira, C., Fitzgerald, N., & Essue, B. (2021, March 15). The Out-of-Pocket Cost Burden of Cancer Care—A Systematic Literature Review. Current Oncology. https://doi.org/10.3390/curroncol28020117

Peh, W. (2021, October 4). Peer review: concepts, variants and controversies. Singapore Medical Journal. https://doi.org/10.11622/smedj.2021139

Smith, R. (2006, April 1). Peer review: a flawed process at the heart of science and journals. Journal of the Royal Society of Medicine. https://doi.org/10.1258/jrsm.99.4.178

There Are Failures, You Know. (2021). Science.org. https://doi.org/10.1126/blog-post.12472

Toscano, F., Vera, A., Kim, E., Golinelli, D., Vila-Reyes, H., Bteich, F., Schernberg, A., Seban, R.-D., Yeh, R., & Dercle, L. (2021, August 25). The Role of Cost-Effectiveness Analysis in Patient-Centered Cancer Care in the Era of Precision Medicine. Cancers. https://doi.org/10.3390/cancers13174272

Women's health concerns are dismissed more, studied less. (2019, December 17). Magazine. https://www.nationalgeographic.com/magazine/article/womens-health-concerns-are-dismissed-more-studied-less-feature

**Chapter 8 The Pattern of Suppression**

Chopra, S. S. (2003, July 2). Industry Funding of Clinical Trials: Benefit or Bias? JAMA. https://doi.org/10.1001/jama.290.1.113

Fønnebø, V., Grimsgaard, S., Walach, H., Ritenbaugh, C., Norheim, A. J., MacPherson, H., Lewith, G., Launsø, L., Koithan, M., Falkenberg, T., Boon, H., & Aickin, M. (2007, February 11). Researching complementary and alternative treatments – the gatekeepers are not at home. BMC Medical Research Methodology. https://doi.org/10.1186/1471-2288-7-7

Herman, P. M., Craig, B. M., & Caspi, O. (2005, June 2). Is complementary and alternative medicine (CAM) cost-effective? a systematic review. BMC Complementary and Alternative Medicine. https://doi.org/10.1186/1472-6882-5-11

Lexchin, J. (2003, May 29). Pharmaceutical industry sponsorship and research outcome and quality: systematic review. BMJ. https://doi.org/10.1136/bmj.326.7400.1167

Mortada, E. (2024). Evidence-Based Complementary and Alternative Medicine in Current Medical Practice. Cureus. https://doi.org/10.7759/cureus.52041

Ross, C. L. (2009, January). Article Commentary: Integral Healthcare: The Benefits and Challenges of Integrating Complementary and Alternative Medicine with a Conventional Healthcare Practice. Integrative Medicine Insights. https://doi.org/10.4137/imi.s2239

Ventola, C. L. (2010, August). Current Issues Regarding Complementary and Alternative Medicine (CAM) in the United States: Part 1: The Widespread Use of CAM and the Need for Better-Informed Health Care Professionals to Provide Patient Counseling. Pharmacy and Therapeutics. https://pmc.ncbi.nlm.nih.gov/articles/PMC2935644/

**Chapter 9 RFK, Autism, and the War on Truth**

Bukar, A. (2020). The Political Economy of Hate Industry: Islamophobia in the Western Public Sphere. Islamophobia Studies Journal. https://doi.org/10.13169/islastudj.5.2.0152

Baweja, R., Brown, S. L., Edwards, E. M., & Murray, M. J. (2021, March 10). COVID-19 Pandemic and Impact on Patients with Autism Spectrum Disorder. Journal of Autism and Developmental Disorders. https://doi.org/10.1007/s10803-021-04950-9

Dal Pai, J., Wolff, C. G., Aranchipe, C. S., Kepler, C. K., Dos Santos, G. A., Canton, L. A. L., de Carvalho, A. B., Richter, S. A., & Nunes, M. L. (2022, September 23). COVID-19 Pandemic and Autism Spectrum Disorder, Consequences to Children and Adolescents - a Systematic Review. Review Journal of Autism and Developmental Disorders. https://doi.org/10.1007/s40489-022-00344-4

Igyártó, B. Z., & Qin, Z. (2024). The mRNA-LNP vaccines - the good, the bad and the ugly? Frontiers in Immunology. https://doi.org/10.3389/fimmu.2024.1336906

Nash, E. J. (2018, June). In Defense of "Targeting" Some Dissent about Science. Perspectives on Science. https://doi.org/10.1162/posc_a_00277

Schindler, S. (2015, April). Architectural Exclusion: Discrimination and Segregation Through Physical Design of the Built Environment. Www.yalelawjournal.org. https://www.yalelawjournal.org/article/architectural-exclusion

Wallis, V. (2023, April 25). The Impact of Censorship on Covid-19 Policy Formation in the United States. Medical Research Archives. https://doi.org/10.18103/mra.v11i4.3822

de Melo-Martín, I., & Intemann, K. (2012, February 8). Scientific dissent and public policy. EMBO Reports. https://doi.org/10.1038/embor.2013.8

**Chapter 10 The Uncomfortable Truth About Medicine**

Georgetown University. (2019). Disease Management Programs: Improving health while reducing costs? - Health Policy Institute. Health Policy Institute. https://hpi.georgetown.edu/management/

History. (2021). Bayer.com. https://www.bayer.com/en/history/1925-1945

Holman, H. R. (2020). The Relation of the Chronic Disease Epidemic to the Health Care Crisis. ACR Open Rheumatology. https://doi.org/10.1002/acr2.11114

Meller, A., & Ahmed, H. (2019, August 30). How Big Pharma Reaps Profits While Hurting Everyday Americans. Center for American Progress. https://www.americanprogress.org/article/big-pharma-reaps-profits-hurting-everyday-americans/

Skender, B. (2024, August 22). The demise of the antibiotic pipeline: the Bayer case. Humanities and Social Sciences Communications; Palgrave Macmillan. https://doi.org/10.1057/s41599-024-03584-3

Text - H.R.1865 - 116th Congress (2019-2020): Further Consolidated Appropriations Act, 2020. (2019). Congress.gov. https://www.congress.gov/bill/116th-congress/house-bill/1865/text

Woodcock, J. (2019, November 1). Safeguarding Pharmaceutical Supply Chains in a Global Economy - 10/30/2019. FDA. https://www.fda.gov/news-events/congressional-testimony/safeguarding-pharmaceutical-supply-chains-global-economy-10302019

Zahr, N. M., Mayer, D., Rohlfing, T., Hasak, M. P., Hsu, O., Vinco, S., Orduna, J., Luong, R., Sullivan, E. V., & Adolf Pfefferbaum. (2010, May

1). Brain Injury and Recovery Following Binge Ethanol: Evidence from In Vivo Magnetic Resonance Spectroscopy. Biological Psychiatry; Elsevier BV. https://doi.org/10.1016/j.biopsych.2009.10.028

**Chapter 11 a Legacy They Couldn't Kill**

Andrew, S. (2023, October 4). Book bans are surging — and taking an emotional toll on many authors. CNN. https://www.cnn.com/2023/10/04/style/book-bans-sales-authors-impact-cec/index.html

BookBaker. (2024). BookBaker. https://www.bookbaker.com/en/v/The-Evolution-of-YouTube-A-Study-of-Youtubers-and-Online-Culture-YouTubes-Impact-on-Traditional-Media/8a0e04a7-13ec-4166-9dc4-fa57b0112599/6

Is YouTube a Good Choice for Your Video Business? (2024, April 8). Gumlet. https://www.gumlet.com/learn/youtube-for-business/

Meehan, K. (2024, November 1). Banned in the USA: Beyond the Shelves. PEN America; PEN America. https://pen.org/report/beyond-the-shelves/

Martinez, N., Connelly, C., Perez, A., & Calero, P. (2021). Self-care: A concept analysis. International Journal of Nursing Sciences. https://doi.org/10.1016/j.ijnss.2021.08.007

Oksanen, A., Celuch, M., Oksa, R., & Savolainen, I. (2024, August 2). Online communities come with real-world consequences for individuals and societies. Communications Psychology. https://doi.org/10.1038/s44271-024-00112-6

Paterick, T. E., Patel, N., Tajik, A. J., & Chandrasekaran, K. (2017). Improving health outcomes through patient education and partnerships with patients. Baylor University Medical Center Proceedings; National Library of Medicine. https://doi.org/10.1080/08998280.2017.11929552

Salleh, S. M., Yusof, H. S. M., Mohammed, N. H., Zahari, A. S. M., & Hamzah, S. F. M. (2020, April 1). Knowledge Sharing in Online Community: A Review. Journal of Physics: Conference Series. https://doi.org/10.1088/1742-6596/1529/2/022052

**Chapter 12 What They Don't Want You to Know**

Alnuqaydan, A. M. (2024, August 26). The dark side of beauty: an in-depth analysis of the health hazards and toxicological impact of synthetic cosmetics and personal care products. Frontiers in Public Health; Frontiers Media. https://doi.org/10.3389/fpubh.2024.1439027

Liu, Z., Yang, R., Chen, H., & Zhang, X. (2025, March 24). Recent Advances in Food Safety: Nanostructure-Sensitized Surface-Enhanced Raman Sensing. Foods; MDPI AG. https://doi.org/10.3390/foods14071115

Swiss Company Charged by FTC with Making Unsubstantiated Health Claims. (2003, January 27). Federal Trade Commission. https://www.ftc.gov/news-events/news/press-releases/2003/01/swiss-company-charged-ftc-making-unsubstantiated-health-claims

Schmalz, G., Falk Schwendicke, Hickel, R., & Platt, J. A. (2023, December 1). Alternative Direct Restorative Materials for Dental Amalgam: A Concise Review Based on an FDI Policy Statement. International Dental Journal; Elsevier BV. https://doi.org/10.1016/j.identj.2023.11.004

The Cornucopia Institute. (2016, August 16). Report Finds Toxins/Carcinogens in Popular Brands of Toothpaste - Cornucopia Institute. Cornucopia Institute. https://www.cornucopia.org/2016/08/report-finds-toxinscarcinogens-in-popular-brands-of-toothpaste/

Team, O. (2008, February 13). Top 10: Quackiest Quacks. OncLive. https://www.onclive.com/view/top10quacks

Woods, J. O. (2015, February). Dr Hal Alan Huggins, Noted Dental Pioneer, Passes Away. Integrative Medicine: A Clinician's Journal. https://pmc.ncbi.nlm.nih.gov/articles/PMC4566458/

Walraven, T., Busch, M., Wang, J., Donkers, J. M., Marjolijn Duijvestein, Evita, Kramer, N. I., & Bouwmeester, H. (2024, September 9). Elevated risk of adverse effects from foodborne contaminants and drugs in inflammatory bowel disease: a review. Archives of Toxicology; Springer Science+Business Media. https://doi.org/10.1007/s00204-024-03844-w

## Don't miss out!

Visit the website below and you can sign up to receive emails whenever Wayne C. Robinson publishes a new book. There's no charge and no obligation.

https://books2read.com/r/B-A-TOYXD-MIERG

Connecting independent readers to independent writers.

Did you love *The Hulda Clark Story*? Then you should read *Silenced Healers: Dr. Hulda Clark, and Others Who Were Silenced*[1] by Wayne C. Robinson!

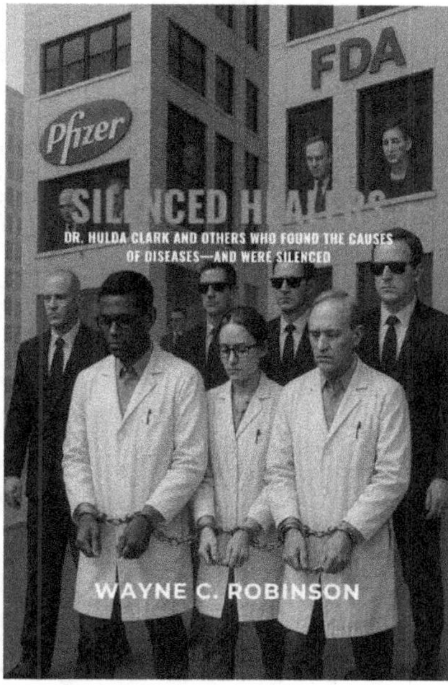

[2]

*The Untold Stories of Rife, Clark, and Sebi—Silenced Voices Who Dared to Heal.*

Why do so many diseases remain "incurable"? Why are powerful, natural treatments buried while pharmaceutical giants thrive? In *Suppressed Healers*, uncover the gripping true stories of three controversial pioneers—Dr. Royal Rife, Dr. Hulda Clark, and Dr. Sebi—who each claimed to discover the hidden causes of disease and, more importantly, how to heal them.

Their groundbreaking research challenged the medical establishment—and the establishment fought back. Branded as frauds, ridiculed by the media, and targeted by authorities, these healers paid a steep price for daring to question the status quo.

This eye-opening book reveals:

The shocking discoveries each scientist made about the root causes of diseases like cancer, AIDS, and chronic illnesses.The systematic suppression that kept

---

1. https://books2read.com/u/m0LvxJ

2. https://books2read.com/u/m0LvxJ

their findings from reaching the public.The powerful role of pharmaceutical profits, media manipulation, and institutional control in silencing alternative healing.How their legacies are quietly living on through those who have taken back control of their health.

*Suppressed Healers* isn't just a history lesson—it's a call to question, to research, and to reclaim your power over your own body. If you've ever wondered why true cures remain hidden, this book holds the key to understanding the forces that shape modern medicine—and how you can break free.

Read more at www.enemieswithinus.com.

# Also by Wayne C. Robinson

**Enemies Within Us**
The Hulda Clark Story
Silenced Healers: Dr. Hulda Clark, and Others Who Were Silenced
The USAID Scandal: How Billions Disappeared
Why Black Americans No Longer Need DEI
USAID And Child Trafficking
COVID 19 Lawsuits
America is $37 Trillion in Debt
Unfit to lead– The End of The Democratic Party
Black Fatigue
The Red Shift
The 2025 Real State of Black America
Die Hulda Clark Story
The Job Hunt is a Scam: Here's How to Beat It
The Sanctuary City Scam And Black Americans
The Global Black MLM Trap
2026 The Year the Democratic Party Collapses
The Global Black MLM/Networking Marketing Trap
Faith, Migration & Power

**Everything About Timeshares**
Cancel Your Timeshare Today
Everything About Timeshares (2025 Edition)

Watch for more at www.enemieswithinus.com.

www.ingramcontent.com/pod-product-compliance
Lightning Source LLC
LaVergne TN
LVHW052258200926
848481LV00002B/400